7 days
to a
slimmer
you

MICHELE
SIMMONS

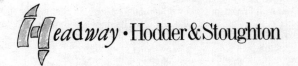

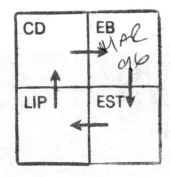

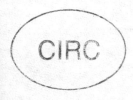

Cataloguing in Publication Data is available from the British Library

ISBN 0 340 595116

First published 1994
Impression number 10 9 8 7 6 5 4 3 2
Year   1999 1998 1997 1996 1995 1994

Typeset by Wearset, Boldon, Tyne and Wear.
Printed in Great Britain for Hodder & Stoughton Educational, a division of Hodder Headline Plc, Mill Road, Dunton Green, Sevenoaks, Kent TN13 2YA by Cox & Wyman Limited, Reading.

CONTENTS

ACKNOWLEDGEMENTS

I would like to thank Dr Sue Jebb at the Dunn Nutrition Centre for her help in checking some of my copy (and so quickly!) as well as Dr Nigel Dickie, Nutrition Consultant to Heinz Weight Watchers, whose vast experience of slimming was invaluable. I am also grateful to the Sports Council for taking the time to go through the exercise chapter. My thanks, too, to nutritionist Amanda Ursell (and her computer!) for so meticulously checking my calories and uncomplainingly converting my ounces to grams, and back again!

I'd also like to thank everyone who has supported, listened, advised and calmed me throughout all the time it has taken to write this book. In particular, Chris McLaughlin, who listened, read and reassured me, Sue Phipps, who gave me the confidence to actually write this in the first place, and Lilian Cordell, who patiently tasted, adjusted and cooked – all in the name of being neighbourly! Most of all though, I thank Jeff Ostrove, for his relentless support, help – and love. I couldn't have done it without him.

INTRODUCTION

Could you do with losing weight but hate the whole idea of slimming? If you could, then the chances are this isn't the first diet book you've picked up. And if that's the case, it means that every other diet you have tried to follow has well and truly let you down. But, you may be surprised to learn that you're not alone because, according to the experts, there's an awful lot of us around who simply don't seem able to stick to a diet successfully. But why?

It's my firm belief that up to now, most diets have borne little or no resemblance to reality or the lives we *really* lead; at the same time, so many slimming programmes are based on a philosophy geared towards making a slimmer feel that to break a diet is to have sinned indeed. However, the explanation for dieting disasters doesn't stop there.

THE CASE AGAINST DIETING

One of the reasons people *don't* stick to diets is because, in many cases, they're downright boring. Food should be one of the joys of life, and not surprisingly, considering that taste is one of our basic senses. Admittedly not every meal can be a gastronomic adventure, but most should at least be greeted with some degree of excited anticipation. If, however, your day's intake consists only of food that's 'wholesome', or looks and tastes like rabbit food, or is so full of fibre that it fills your stomach but leaves your mouth craving for chocolate, then you shouldn't be surprised that you never reach the end of the diet sheet – or book!

We need variety when it comes to food and we need to feel that we've enjoyed what we've eaten. Without the enjoyment factor every diet is doomed to failure because you end up with a dissatisfied stomach, and dissatisfied stomachs lead to night-time nibbling or, even worse, a diet in tatters and a waistline that just seems to grow . . . and grow, and one very disappointed *ex*-dieter.

Which leads me on to another reason why we *don't* stick to diets. People want a change. Sometimes we just don't fancy yet another week of the same meals as the last, with the same recipes, the same amounts and following the same formula. What's more, given half the chance, we want food to suit our mood. It would be a very single-minded person indeed who would be content with cottage cheese salad and weak tea (no milk!) every day. After all, if it's cold it's only natural that we want something hot to warm us through and make us feel satisfied inside as well as out.

Also, there are times when we simply aren't in the mood to stand over a stove steaming our vegetables while our four ounces of skinless chicken dry-roasts in the oven. Yes, admittedly there are plenty of low-fat cookery books and slimming recipes around that can teach the rudiments of good cooking the healthy way but often the dishes take a good deal of thought and preparation to conjure up and they need patience, application and *time*. You've also got to feel in the *mood* for *cordon bleu* – low-cal. or otherwise – something that is rare for most of us to feel all of the time or, for that matter, all of us to feel most of the time.

◆THE LONELINESS OF THE LONG DISTANCE SLIMMER

Another reason people don't stick to diets is because they can be anti-social. Flatmates, partners and offspring invariably don't see quite the attraction in the low-calorie dishes that you do. So, you either end up making several, separate meals each day or you decide to eat by yourself, if only to avoid the callous comments from the people you live with about the excuse for food that is unhappily nestling in the corner of your plate.

And have you ever tried going out to eat with friends when you're trying to stick to your diet? If you're taking your diet seriously the only way you can consider eating anything is by prefacing your order with a barrage of questions – 'No butter with my bread, unless of course you have some low-fat, polyunsaturated margarine?' And then there's what to eat – grilled fish is usually fairly safe but 'Has it been basted in butter *before* it's been grilled?'.

You either spend the evening questioning the waiter about how things are cooked – animal fat, vegetable fat, no fat? – or you meekly order a little something from the side-salad section, trying hard to control your excitement when the waiter returns from the kitchen to tell you that the cook has offered to turn your order of mixed lettuces, garnished with fresh parsley and black pepper, from a side-dish into a full-blown, main course! Your host congratulates the cook on his imagination and initiative; you, on the other hand, sit fantasising about *pasta carbonara* followed by chocolate mousse, lashings of cream and a plate of *petits fours* . . .

Most diets also fail due to their sheer magnitude: they always seem such a long-term commitment! The idea of sticking to any diet that's based on eating exactly the same foods for weeks on end is bound to put all but the most single-minded off. And having to plan anything that runs into months is often too vast to contemplate. It's also restrictive because it means you become wary of making arrangements for the future in case the plans don't fit into your food schedule. But, when you are pushed into making plans that involve eating out, what do you do? I'll tell you what – invariably you say, 'Stuff the diet!', enjoy the fun and – nine times out of ten – spend the evening in question eating everything in sight. Nobody, but nobody, likes to think that they *have* to stick to anything for weeks on end, particularly when that something is based on deprivation, deprivation that only affects you, when those all around are happily enjoying the pleasures of the food of their choice, blissfully unaware of the untold suffering of one so near. No wonder so many women find it easier to be successful sinners rather than successful slimmers!

But it needn't be so. It's my belief that if, up to now, you have been an unsuccessful slimmer, for any, or all, of the reasons I've outlined above, it is the diet that has failed – not you. Diets don't *have* to be boring, or anti-social, restrictive, time-consuming or based on deprivation. There is another way and *7 Days to a Slimmer You* is *it*.

In this diet, each week's food plan is looked at as a group of seven days. I ask you to plan no further in advance than that. What I can guarantee, though, is that at the end of every seven days you'll discover a slimmer you. Obviously, the more seven-day eating plans you follow, the more you lose, but the decision over how many diets you try – and how often – is up to you.

What's more, this whole book takes into account your mood, your taste, your family and even your lifestyle. And the good news is, that no-one expects you to spend hours preparing each meal or shopping for weird and wonderful ingredients that may well be as good for your body as they are for your waistline but the likelihood is that they're hard to find, and once you do track them down you find they're expensive, difficult to use and you have to buy a kilo when you only need a couple of teaspoons!

▼IVE LA DIFFÉRENCE!

This diet is different to all other diets because it takes into account *who* you are as well as *what* you are. It realises that you may have a family to cook for, friends to eat out with and often not much time – or inclination – to slave away at a hot stove. This is also the first diet that *doesn't* assume that meat and two veg. is everyone's choice for a main meal or that everyone has time to make themselves lunch as well as preparing a family meal in the evening. The diet works from the basis that, particularly during the week, most people have a rushed breakfast and a hastily eaten snack for lunch which is often consumed while doing something else at the same time. This diet also recognises the fact that because the first two meals of the day are eaten in such a rush, the chances are that by tea-time you're starving, so the diet has a built-in snack factor, to be eaten when you feel like it and when you've got time.

What's more, because the reality is that people have different tastes and different moods, I've included recipes that do need some preparation as well as others that need virtually none. I've included take-aways (with one survey by the Economist Intelligence Unit revealing that this is the fastest growing food market it would be unrealistic not to) as well as snack meals, dishes for the family, foods for 'thin days' and foods for 'fat days'. There's a section on eating out (if you know what to choose that's half the battle) as well as a chapter that allows for cook-chill foods – when you're buying out to eat in.

By being flexible about what today's dieter can eat, I believe the real joy of *7 Days to a Slimmer You* is that this is a diet that works *for* you and your lifestyle. So, if you want to eat out every night of the week, that's fine, and you can discover exactly how to in chapter 9. Likewise if you want your diet to centre around take-aways or home cooking, you just turn to chapters 11 or 7 respectively. All the diet chapters are designed to be mixed and matched, depending on what you feel like eating and on how much you want to lose. Only you know what sort of weight loss is right for you so it's up to you to decide how long you want to stick to the eating plans.

But, and this is a big *but*, the real beauty of this diet is that if you fancy eating out just once a week, or eating curry, take-away, or cooking at home just once or twice a week, that's fine too. Simply pick one (or two) day's eating plan from the appropriate chapter and then simply mix and match the day(s) you have selected with eating plans from the other chapters. So, if Monday is take-away night, then – depending on the take-away – you choose an eating plan from chapter 11. If the rest of the week is spent at home, you then need chapter 7 where you'll be able to pick six days of menus that can fit into family life. And if by Friday you're happy to settle for something ready-made from the freezer, take a look at some of dieting days in chapter 10, and replace one of these six with your choice.

It's all so easy! All you need do is simply use the chapter index to choose the food to match your mood, your pocket, your taste, or your waistline. You won't find an easier way of getting down to your goal weight and if, in the unlikely event, your weight should start to creep up again, then quickly putting yourself back on one, or all, of the seven-day eating plans will slim you back into shape in no time at all. It really is *that* simple.

So, whether you need a temporary eating plan to help you get back into shape or a long-term strategy to help you to discover *any* shape, this is the book for you. And if you still don't believe that it's possible to eat the foods you like and lose weight, now's your chance to try! All I ask is that you give it seven days, that's all it takes, seven days to discover the road to a slimmer you.

◆ ◆ ◆

1 A LITTLE BIT ABOUT HOW WE LOSE WEIGHT . . .

Now, this is the *easy* bit. It's all about the theory of losing weight and, as I'm sure you know, it's not until you try to put the theory into practice that you run into problems! That said, the more you understand about some of the reasons why we put on weight, the easier it is to start exercising some control over your body. And, yes, it *is* possible to control it and how it behaves.

For the time being, think of your body as a car, with you in the driving seat. Basically, your body relies on food to keep it going – just like a car needs fuel. Once eaten, our food is converted into what scientists call *energy* and this is used by our bodies for circulation, breathing, digestion and generally keeping our bodies ticking over, in the same way as a car engine burns petrol to keep it going. This process of 'filling up' can be called 'input', and is measured in *calories*, a term somewhat more familiar to dieters!

So what do you do with your energy?

We're all used to thinking of calories as baddies because we associate them with calorie-laden foods like gateaux and chocolate bars but actually a calorie is simply a term used for measuring a unit of energy.

Input is, as I've said, what you put into your body in terms of food – and this includes teas, coffees, the odd biscuit at elevenses, the chips the children didn't finish at lunchtime, the slice of bread that was left over from breakfast – in fact, it includes almost everything that passes your lips.

When it comes to food our bodies are actually very democratic because once it's gone into our system, the body shares it out, each organ taking what it needs to keep it going. And, in the same way as a car can only be filled with so much petrol, we too only need a specific amount of food to keep us going. If we eat more than we need, the body has a unique (and some would say rather unfortunate!) way of dealing with it: it sends it to the stores department – or to be more precise, the fat stores department. The idea being that it's kept there for the day when food becomes so scarce that the body has to draw on its reserves, or fat stores, to keep it going. However, these days, food scarcity is rare, which means the calls on our stores department are few and far between, which goes some way to explaining why so many of us are overweight!

Now clearly your body needs energy to keep it going, but as I've explained, there's a limit to how much energy it needs. The actual amount depends on what is known as your 'output', in other words, what you actually *do* with your energy. This takes into account how active you are. It includes any exercise you've had and how much effort you've put into, say, going up the stairs or running for the bus. Even housework counts as output in the energy picture: scrubbing the floor uses up an awful lot more energy than, say, dusting the bedroom.

Everything you do uses energy (even sleeping) because your body constantly needs a certain amount of energy, even if it's just to keep your heart, liver and lungs ticking over. Needless to say, sleeping uses up far fewer calories than something that requires considerably more activity. So, someone who goes swimming three times a week, plays squash twice and goes walking at weekends is going to need more calories a day to stop them losing weight because their output is greater than average. Someone who drives everywhere, considers running for a taxi gross exertion, slumps in front of the TV at night and will only walk up the stairs when it's time to go to bed will clearly have a much smaller output than her sporty friend. Your body is a little like those old-fashioned scales with weighing dishes on each side; the trick is to make both sides balance. Too much on one side and the balance is disturbed.

Your body then has to work out what to do with all the extra food and it has a simple answer – it turns it into fat stores. To lose weight, the scale with the energy you use up has to be heavier than the scale with your day's worth of food and drink.

For our bodies to turn the food into energy, it has to go through a sort of biological conversion process, called 'metabolism'. So, one way or another, everything we eat is 'metabolised'. Now not all of us burn up our energy at the same speed and it's normal for the speed of our metabolism to vary from person to person. In fact, at one stage it was thought that if you were considerably overweight then one of the reasons was that you had a slow metabolism, but subsequent research has revealed the exact opposite: by carrying around all that excess weight your body is forced to work harder, which means that your metabolic rate is faster rather than slower. So the reality is that it's the skinnies who have the metabolism which, on a day-to-day basis, doesn't use up as much energy.

◆WHY METABOLISM MATTERS

However, everyone can boost the amount of energy they use and the most effective way of kick-starting your metabolism is to increase your output, in other words to increase your physical activity. In fact, some experts believe that our energy continues to be burnt up at a faster rate not just while we're being active but also for several hours afterwards. Of course it all depends on the type of activity you're involved in, as well as for how long, but the hard truth is that, when it comes to weight, the more you do, the more you lose!

Now if the very thought of exercise makes you want to lie down in a darkened room, you'll be pleased to know that increasing your output doesn't mean you have to spend every waking hour clad in a leotard (although, of course, a regular exercise class is as good for your shape as it is for your health). The good news is, that all you need to do is spend around 20 minutes, three times a week, doing anything from walking (albeit briskly) to going for a regular swim. Keep-fit, jogging, playing tennis, running or even cycling are all great ways of increasing your output *and* improving your health.

Exercise doesn't have to be a chore, as you can see for yourself in chapter 14. And even if you're one of those people who would rather have teeth pulled than put on a track suit, do at least *read* the chapter. Even if it gets you running up the stairs and walking to the shops, at least it's a start. And it's worth remembering that if you're out there increasing your energy output, be it on the tennis court or in the swimming pool, you're actually removed from the temptations that result in energy input!

♦OOD, GLORIOUS FOOD

Whether you believe in the benefits of exercise or not, if you're an unsuccessful slimmer, then the likeliest cause of your dieting downfall is a four lettered word – *food*. Obviously, it's important to enjoy what we eat, but if food, whether buying it, cooking it or eating it, plays a large part in your life, you might take comfort in the fact that you're not alone. And when it comes to eating it, in particular, it's something of a national pastime. Even a glance at the statistics reveals that, largely, we're a nation of fatties. A recent survey, carried out for the Department of Health revealed that 53 per cent of men and 44 per cent of women were overweight. And the number appears to be increasing.

But why? Obviously a large part of the problem is that our bodies now need less energy than they used to, simply because we *do* less than we used to. The blame for our sedentary lifestyle is largely due, would you believe, to 'progress'! Strange as it may seem, we used to lead much more active lives, even though the people who actually exercised were probably few and far between. Progress has resulted in a multitude of labour-saving devices, all geared towards making our lives easier. For example, most homes now have washing machines, vacuum cleaners, spin dryers (so we don't even need to hang washing out anymore), dishwashers, self-cleaning ovens, while freezers and fridges have cut down the need for a daily shop. Television has assumed greater dominance in all our lives and most of us spend a fair proportion of our week slumped in front of the box. And remote control means you don't need to exert even the energy to change the channel! Cars too come with automatic extras -like those nifty buttons that save our muscles the tedium of opening the window!

Of course I'm not saying that we'd want to go back to washing the sheets in the bath or walking miles every day for a pint of milk or a loaf of bread. But, for our bodies, all this progress has come to mean that we're conserving the energy that, in the past, was used up by everyday tasks. And, as we don't seem to be reducing our food intake accordingly, the result is that we're getting fatter. In fact, experts reckon that we should consume around a third fewer calories than we did 50 years ago, precisely because we expend so much less energy. As our bodies seem to be paying a price for progress, it becomes even more important that we adapt to their new needs – call them the needs of the 90s, if you like. As we've seen, exercise, or increasing your output, can make a huge difference to your weight, particularly if you don't have very much to lose.

EATING BETTER, NOT LESS

Although it's never too late to increase your output, when it comes to actually dieting, the most important element in any weight loss pro-gramme is to adjust your input. But that doesn't necessarily mean that you have to cut right back on food, re-organise mealtimes or radically re-think your eating habits. With a little planning and thought you can have three meals a day, snacks if you fancy them, and still go over to friends for a take-away.

Of course, this doesn't mean that you don't have to make some changes to what you eat – but it is possible to choose a diet to suit your lifestyle, as well as your tastebuds. The most important thing is to make sure you are well-informed enough about food to be able to make the sort of choices that suit your mood and circumstances as well as your body.

A diet that works is not the sort of diet that leaves you hungry or feeling deprived of the foods that you enjoy. To slim successfully, you need a system that allows you to eat the sort of foods that make you feel full *and* satisfied, and for a diet really to work, you need to know you're going to feel good too. Being hungry and not eating the right kinds of food can lead to irritability, lack of energy, apathy and even depression. As we've seen, food provides the energy that keeps our bodies going; without it we initially fail to operate efficiently and can, eventually, fail to operate at all.

THE BALANCING ACT

Healthy eating these days is all about eating the foods that are rich in vitamins and minerals and provide the maximum nutrients that our bodies need to keep them in peak condition. No single food provides all the nutrients we need in the amounts we need them, so it really is essential to eat a mixture of foods that are able to provide the maximum nourishment. The latest thinking stresses the importance of making sure we get a good mixture of proteins (fish, meat and cheese, or vegetable sources such as pulses and cereals), carbohydrates (such as bread and pasta, preferably the unrefined sort) and fruit and vegetables in our diet. It's all a question of balance and it's vital to get the balance right. And it's worth remembering that there's no such thing as a good or bad food; there are only good or bad diets.

Food can largely be divided into three basic groups – protein, carbohydrate and fat – all of which play a crucial part in keeping our bodies working. Protein provides the basic building blocks of the body and is needed for growth and replacement of our cells and tissues. Carbohydrates are a main source of energy for our body, as are fats, although, weight for weight, fats are a much richer source. Fats also provide essential fatty acids (needed for growth and development) as well as helping our bodies process and use the fat-soluble vitamins, A,D,E and K. So it's impossible to have a completely fat-free diet; a small amount of fat is needed by our bodies. That said, it's worth remembering that each gram of fat generates about nine calories, whereas a gram of carbohydrate or protien is worth around four. So, clearly a diet that's high in fat is going to be more likely to make *you* fat. The following seven-day diets offer an eating regime that gives the right sort of balance for you and your body. That way, you end up feeling as good as you look.

The idea of the following pages is to show that you can eat more or less what you want with the minimum of change. All the evidence now emphasises the need to eat more of particular types of food and less of others. So, it really is a case of eating better, rather than less, and also making sure that every calorie is a wanted calorie.

Apart from being rich in vitamins and minerals, your meals will all be low-fat, low-sugar and high in fibre. Low-fat because not only does fat contain more calories than any other type of food, but because high-fat diets (particularly those diets high in saturated, or animal fat) have been found to be a contributory factor in a number of diseases, including coronary heart disease, stroke, some cancers and high blood pressure. However, it's worth mentioning that even though animal fats, which are saturated, are a lot richer than vegetable fats, which are generally unsaturated, all fat is loaded with calories and too many calories lead to excess weight. So, simply reducing the saturated fats in your diet may be better for your heart but unless you reduce *all* the fats in your diet you're still going to find that you're piling on the pounds.

The *7 Days to a Slimmer You* meals are also low in sugar because apart from causing tooth decay, a high intake of sugar may increase your risk of diabetes and even coronary heart disease. Some experts have also blamed 'hidden' sugars for the fact that we've become a nation of fatties. Refined sugar is really a form of 'empty' calories, offering little goodness and containing none of the essential vitamins, minerals or proteins found in other foodstuffs. Unfortunately, though, it isn't easy to cut sugar from your diet as it's used in many savoury foods as well as sweet ones. For example, you may be aware that sweets are the result of bags of sugar combined with drops of food colouring, but did you also realise that spoonfuls of sugar, literally, are added to your tomato ketchup, baked beans, tinned vegetables and tinned soups, as well as a vast selction of savoury frozen foods? Fizzy drinks are full of it too, so a couple of thirst-quenching glasses of sparkling orange can clock up the same amount of calories as a main course meal!

You'll also find many of the meal plans high in fibre, or what used to be called 'roughage'. Foods that are high in fibre include wholegrain cereals, peas, beans, fruit and vegetables. 'Dietary fibre' refers to the fibres that are naturally present in the food that we eat. These foods not only take longer to eat (they're generally more chewy) but they also provide bulk in the diet, which means you feel full, quicker, and so you don't have as much room for fatty foods. Also, high-fibre foods take longer to digest, which means you feel full for longer. But the advantages of a high-fibre diet don't stop there. Fibre-rich foods can help avoid constipation, an irritable colon and even *diverticulitis* (inflammation of the large intestine). It is also thought that certain types of fibre can help reduce cholesterol levels in the blood, therefore reducing the risk of heart disease.

Of course you can try to lose weight without following any of these basic principles. And you may well find a way to lose weight that requires no thought, no planning, no effort and no restrictions. If that's the case, I guarantee that not only will you find that the pounds pile back on (see the next chapter for exactly why) but the chances are you could end up feeling, and being, quite ill. And if you're not actually well enough to enjoy the new, slimmer you – then what's the point? Once this happens, human nature tells us that we end up searching for ways to console ourselves. And guess what's the most common form of consolation? That's right, you guessed it – food! And taking solace in the comfort of food is a guaranteed way of putting the pounds back on – but even more quickly than before – as you'll discover in chapter 2!

◆ ◆ ◆

2 HOW DIETS WORK

According to statistics, 65 per cent of British women and 34 per cent of men are trying to lose weight. Rounded up, that means that at any given time, over nine and a half *million* women, and just under five *million* men, are on a diet, or one-in-four of the population. And the older you get, the more likely you are to slim. So, if this is your first diet then you're in a minority!

However, assuming you're one of the majority, ask yourself exactly how many diets you have tried over the years. Can you remember? And which ones? You have to admit there's been quite a choice. And as each new diet has come along, it's been accompanied by a new theory, depending on what happened to be in vogue at the time. When first introduced, each one always seemed a completely new concept, an answer to a fatty's prayer if you like, always suggesting a miracle 'cure' for weight reduction – the perfect way to peel off the pounds.

Some claimed that the secret of slimming was based on one type of food that held particular fat-burning properties; others concentrated on the exclusion of whole hosts of foods – if not food altogether – with the promise that all excess weight would disappear, leaving you slimmer, happier, healthier, fat-free – a person who never need say 'diet' again. Which is exactly what may have happened, until you started eating normally again when the pounds simply piled back on. So, you ended up disappointed, disillusioned . . . and still overweight.

When you think about it, over the years we've been confused by carbohydrates, blinded by protein, bamboozled by brown fat, enticed by enzymes and even learnt to love the occasional meal in a glass. At the time, the basis of each diet seems so very different but the truth of the matter is that, apart from centring around either gimmicks or gurus, they all have one thing in common. The unlikely link? It's simple once you think about it – they don't work!

◆WHY THEY DON'T WORK

The reason for this, however, is no secret. They don't work because not only do the eating regimes bear no resemblance to the way we really eat but many of them revolve around monotonous or unpalatable meals that are often nutritionally unbalanced. They don't teach anyone anything about sensible eating habits and some even have the added disadvantage of having considerable side-effects, ranging from hunger, bowel problems or indigestion to causing metabolic malfunctioning. Some cause loss of muscle tissue (which you don't want) while others could be potentially harmful, due to loss of tissue protein and body fluid. And, it's worth mentioning that diets based on severe food restrictions can leave you nutritionally deficient, which could end up threatening your general state of health.

You then also have to think about exactly how a severe restriction of food can affect the way your body works. It can be quite dramatic and it's all mainly down to our old friend *metabolism*. What happens when you cut your daily intake of food drastically is that your body goes into a sort of starvation mode and everything slows down in an effort to conserve energy. If you've ever gone without food for a couple of days, either out of choice or because you've lost your appetite through illness, you'll know how light-headed and weak you can feel. And that's because your body has been denied the energy it requires to function. It retaliates by 'slowing down'. This manifests itself in sluggishness and an inability to do anything other than that which requires the bare minimum of energy.

As a result, your body and all its functions – the vital organs, cell replacement and so on – adapt to existing on less energy by drawing on their stores as, ultimately, your body is geared towards helping you survive. So, yes, you do lose weight. However, the bad news is that once you return to your former eating habits, (the ones that caused you to put on weight in the first place), you'll put it all back on again. By adopting a very low-calorie diet you end up working against your body which is trying to save the fat you're trying to get rid of. And sadly I have to tell you that the odds are not in your favour! You may lose weight initially but it'll only be a temporary weight loss, and the more often you put your body under the gruelling regime of a severely restricted diet, the more temporary that loss will be.

In fact, if anything, as your weight goes up and down you start to affect your body's ability to cope with a normal supply of food because you keep sending it mixed messages. As your body learns to cope with less energy your whole metabolism shifts gear. So, the only thing you can be sure of when you lose weight fast is that you'll put it on equally fast. Once you stop eating a restricted diet the pounds start to pile back on again, but this time as fat rather than the muscle that you have lost.

At this point it's also worth considering the original concept behind very low-calorie diets. When they were first introduced their usage was restricted to clinical conditions, for example, in hospital. They were seen as an effective way of controlling extreme *obesity* (that is when people's weight is considered a grave threat to their health). By using these diets in a controlled situation, doctors were able to monitor the effect that a severely restricted diet had on an individual. Also, as the patients were in hospital, they weren't expected to expend much energy and if they felt weak or light headed they could simply take to their beds. No-one expected them to carry out a day's work and if they weren't able to function normally it simply didn't matter.

So, the VLCDs (very low-calorie diets) were never originally intended to be used by the general public; they were intended for use by very overweight people, under medical supervision. They were never seen as a long-term solution to a weight problem.

THE EXPERT VIEW

If there is one thing that the experts *do* agree on it's that the only way to achieve permanent weight loss is to lose the weight steadily over a period of time (the actual period depends on how much you have to lose). Admittedly, it would be wonderful to shed those excess pounds overnight but when you consider that it probably took months, or even years, to put the weight on in the first place, you're going to have to accept that it is going to take a little time to lose it! And, if you do lose weight slowly and change your eating habits, you'll be much more likely to keep the weight off once you've reached your goal. Also, a slower weight loss is more likely to eat into your fat stores, which of course is the object of the exercise.

As we've seen, losing weight does not necessarily mean losing fat. The wrong kind of diet can mean you're losing body fluid which is all too easily replaced, usually simply by having a drink, even if that drink's a glass of water. So, you have to make sure that your new eating plan is really going to suit you and your lifestyle. You also have to be sure that you understand some of the basic principles of weight loss.

The history of slimming has been full of diets based on excluding particular foods, depending on what happens to be in vogue at the time. However, such eating regimes work on the principle of excluding essential nutrients, all of which provide vital fuel for the smooth running of our body. The key to successful slimming is making sure you're getting all the essential nutrients from your diet, while cutting down on the non-essential ones.

WHAT WE ACTUALLY NEED

As we saw in chapter 1, as a nation we're now using a lot less energy than our grandparents, or even our parents, which means we need to take in less energy or, if you prefer, fewer calories.

While the average woman's energy requirement is around 1900 calories a day (for men it is about 600 more) this figure is only approximate because, as we've seen, the number of calories you'll use up, depends on how active you are. Obviously the less you eat, the more you lose, but what we're trying to do here is to get you to eat the sort of foods that mean you can be sure of three things:

◆ that you're getting all the nutrients you need;
◆ that your metabolism can cope with the weight loss effectively; and
◆ that you feel satisfied, full and well.

The third point is the most important factor in a succesful diet plan. Eating is something you should look forward to; it should become an enjoyable part of your life, but not the most important part. So, it's crucial that for any diet to work it has to suit your lifestyle as well as your tastebuds. If the diet you're following means you can't eat with friends and isn't satisfying you then you're simply not going to stick to it. All the odds are against you. It may work for a while, but how long can you last making two meals a day (one for you, one for everyone else) and refusing dinner invitations?

However, to be successful, choosing the diet that suits your tastes as much as your lifestyle *must* involve some changes to your existing eating habits; the secret is to do it so slowly that your appetite and tastebuds don't even notice! Think of it this way: losing weight is not so much about being careful as it is about being clever. And the cleverer you are, the less careful you need to be!

THE SMART WAY TO SLIM

Obviously the last thing anyone wants is to sacrifice all the foods they love, but there are ways of dramatically slashing the calorie-content of some of your favourite foods. *Spaghetti carbonara* doesn't instantly spring to mind as a slimmers' staple (and it's hardly surprising with all that cream, oil, bacon and cheese) and the traditional version can notch up almost 1000 calories, just over half a day's worth of your recommended daily intake! But with a little planning and a dash of culinary skill, the astronomically high dish can be reduced by over half. And the same is true of steak and kidney pie. Or bread and butter pudding. Or ... well, you don't need to take my word for it; once you start the diet you'll soon see for yourself!

Being clever when it comes to calories is all about getting to know about 'alternatives', the dieting goodies. These are the low-fat, low-sugar foods that can turn even the most calorie-loaded meal into a slimmers' friend. And if you're wondering how, the answer lies in one word – 'substitution'.

THE 'NO DIET' APPROACH TO A SLIMMER YOU

These days the supermarket shelves are groaning with low-fat, reduced-sugar and high-fibre goodies. So much so, that slimming has never been easier. Admittedly when some of the earlier low-fat products were launched they were somewhat tough on the digestion and poor on the palate, but we really have come a long way since slimming cheeses tasted distinctly soapy and sweetners fizzed with aftertaste. Now, product for product, it's often hard to tell what's high-fat and what's low-fat. And used in cooking, many 'alternatives' take on a guise that would fool the skills of even the most creative cook. To give you a flavour of what's on offer, the following is a selection of some of the low-calorie foods available from most supermarkets:

- cheeses (from Cheddar to Red Leicester to Brie to cheese spread to cream cheese)
- milk (fresh, long-life), cream (double as well as single!),
- salad dressings, oil-free dressings, mayonnaise, pickle, ketchup
- lean mince (lamb, turkey and beef), low-fat beefburgers, sausages, garlic sausage, bacon
- tinned fish in brine, vegetables in water, fruit in natural juice
- yoghurts, fromage frais, mousses, dairy desserts, frozen yoghurt, ice-cream, ice-cream alternatives, sorbets, jelly, rice pudding
- sugar-free breakfast cereal
- margarines, low-fat spreads, jams, fruit spreads, marmalades
- soups, pâtés, sandwiches, prepared salads, dips
- tinned spaghetti, baked beans
- an absolutely enormous range of cook-chill meals (anything from Prawn Curry and Chicken and Asparagus Bake to Vegetable Lasagne and Cottage Pie)
- fizzy drinks, squashes, sachets of chocolate drinks

The list is almost endless, and I hope it shows that if you really are serious about dieting, finding low-calorie foods to suit your taste should be no problem, regardless of whether you're a meat and two veg. sort of person or you're more partial to the delicacies of *nouvelle cuisine*. Getting to know your healthier options means that when it comes to food, you can have choice and *still* lose weight. The secret is to understand enough about food to be able to make the right choices.

ideally, you want to fill up on foods that give you maximum nourishment with minimum calories. So, we're talking about the 'superfoods' – the ones that are packed with vitamins and minerals but free from the excessive calories which come from too much fat and sugar. Fresh fruit and vegetables are good examples, as are fibre-rich foods such as wholegrain products, like wholemeal bread and pasta and brown rice. The more informed you are, the more chance there is you'll opt for healthier alternatives.

Once you realise that a bag of chocolates can contain as many calories as a main meal – but with none of the nutritional advantages – you may find they seem somewhat less appetising, so you need to be able to recognise the foods that you should steer clear of – the ones that are full of calories but offer nothing in the nourishment stakes. For example, take a typical chocolate bar, like a Mars bar. For your 330 or so calories you get no fibre, no vitamins, possibly some trace minerals and a smidgin of protein. What you *do* get for all those calories is an awful lot of fat. And sugar. And, if you really are that hungry, next time you reach for a Mars bar – or any other bar for that matter – think about what else you can eat for the same number of calories – like five-and-a-half apples, or a cup of soup, a tuna sandwich *and* a yoghurt, or maybe Chicken Chasseur followed by a fruit salad . . . and now ask yourself, honestly, if you're looking for nourishment, is that chocolate bar really such good value?

Chocolate bars, biscuits or packets of sweets all contain what nutritionists call 'empty' calories. They give your body virtually no nourishment in return for large quantities of calories, which can encourage obesity as well as reducing your appetite for other foods which are more nutritionally balanced. So, the important thing to do is to make sure that you eat nutritionally dense foods that give your body what it needs. These foods are also more likely to give you a feeling of fullness which will last at least until your next meal time. And by eating nutritionally dense foods, you won't need to go searching for chocolate bars; you simply won't have the room for them! Just by cutting back on the nutritionally poor, calorie-rich foods you should start to see a difference on the scales in no time. But once you actually start using the seven-day slim plan menus, your weight will start to fall away.

◆ HOW MUCH WILL YOU LOSE?

This depends on how much you have to lose and on how effective your metabolism is. Generally though, scientists have worked out that to lose, say one pound of weight a week, you need to eat around 500 calories fewer than your daily energy requirement. As most of the menu plans amount to anything from just under 1000 to 1200 calories, you should lose about ten pounds in the first month. You'll probably average about two or three pounds a week but you could find you lose anything up to five pounds in the first week. This is due to the loss of *glycogen*, a carbohydrate which is stored in the liver and muscle. When this is lost, water is also shed – hence a good weight loss in the first week or two.

Bear in mind, too, that at certain times in a woman's menstrual cycle she is likely to retain fluid, which could mean a gain of anything from two to seven pounds just before a period. However, although your weight may well seem erratic at these times, you should find that the scales register a significant loss after about a week. So, if your weight loss timetable isn't going to plan, don't give up. There's probably a perfectly sensible explanation and your weight will more than likely balance itself out by the next time you weigh yourself.

You may feel that losing up to three pounds a week isn't enough and you'll get frustrated while you wait to shrink to what you feel is a more appropriate size. If that's the case you need to know a little bit about motivation, which will be revealed in the next chapter. Meanwhile, next time you look in the mirror and feel disappointed because the visible changes just don't seem great enough, take comfort in all the changes that are happening, right there and then, which you can't see. Think of it this way, the longer that you stay overweight and carry around that excess weight, the more chance there is of it having an adverse effect on your health. You increase your risk of suffering from heart disease, high blood pressure, strokes, arthritis, diabetes and some cancers. And it isn't just the life-threatening conditions that make doctors view obesity as a clinical condition. There are many less serious, but none the less miserable conditions that are either caused or aggravated by being overweight: gallstones, constipation, piles, varicose veins – and these are just physical complaints. Apart from lack of confidence and low self-esteem, you may be more prone to depression as well as finding it difficult to keep up with your kids.

The mental torture of feeling severely overweight should never be underestimated. I remember working on a slimming magazine where one of my main jobs was to interview our successful slimmers – women who had lost a substantial amount of weight. To say these women were glowing was an understatement. They radiated pride and success. They had taken control of their lives and succeeded.

However, the stories they told of their former, fatter selves were, at times, heartbreaking.

I remember one woman who couldn't get down on the floor to play with her baby because she knew she wasn't able to get up again. Another who hated walking, not just because it required a huge effort to lug her weight around, although she admitted it did, but because her legs were so large that walking made them rub together and by the time she got home her skin had rubbed so badly her legs were red raw. Another, who when she complained to her husband that they never made love anymore, was told that it was too difficult because she was so big he couldn't get his arms round her. And then there's the more common complaints – 'People always thought I was pregnant' and 'Have you thought of the maternity department for something more your size?' – buying clothes through mail order so you don't have to bare your body in a crowded changing room – or hearing your children's friends asking 'Why's your mum so fat?'

The examples of the psychological pressures of being overweight are endless, as are the examples of the health risks. And when you *do* get a day when your willpower is starting to flag, it's worth reminding yourself that the benefits of losing weight that you can't see are just as great as the benefits that you can.

◆ ◆ ◆

3 A STRATEGY FOR SUCCESSFUL SLIMMING

Now you know a little about how your body works, the next step is to make sure that your mind, or at very least your appetite, is working with your body, rather than against it. Being serious and determined about losing weight really is half the battle. If you're slimming simply because someone else thinks you ought to be, then the diet will be doomed to failure before you've chopped up your first fruit salad or mixed your first oil-free dressing. In fact, trying to slim can be a little like trying to give up smoking. If you don't really want to do it, no amount of cajoling from friends, nagging from family or time spent reading up on why you should give up will make the slightest difference. Whether or not you really want to lose weight is all down to you.

So, if you're not serious, stop reading right here! If, on the other hand, you are, you should know that one of the first requirements for successful slimming is honesty. You need to be totally honest about food; what you eat, what you want to eat and when you eat it. There's no point in cheating because at the end of the day the only person you really cheat is you. Kidding yourself that a couple of biscuits don't count as you graze your way through the pack with a cup of tea while you're waiting for the kids to come home, or watching TV, will do as little for your self-esteem as it will for your diet. The 'odd' biscuit *does* count, as much as the 'odd' roast potato or 'odd' bag of crisps. And if you don't believe me, next time you eat the 'odd' something, just stand on the scales for proof of exactly *how much* it counts.

How much to lose?

You may have found out already that trying to discover the weight you *should* be is something of an inexact science.

Because we're built differently, some of us have a large bone structure; others may be relatively petite. The experts offer a range of weights that are acceptable for someone of a specific height. You've probably looked at these height and weight charts a hundred times, telling yourself that it's okay because you are actually *just* in the acceptable weight range for someone of your height, even though you know you'd be far happier being at the other end of the range!

If you find the charts aren't specific enough for you then a more mathematical way of telling whether you have excess weight is given by your 'body mass index' (BMI). This figure is calculated as follows: weight divided by height, squared. So, weigh yourself in kilograms, then measure your height in metres. Now make the calculation, which is:

$$\frac{\text{weight in kilograms}}{\text{height in metres} \times \text{height in metres}}$$

For both men and women a BMI figure of between 20 and 25 is healthy – over 30 you could be seriously endangering your health.

For example, say you weigh 89 kilos (about 14 stone) and you're 1.7 metres (about 5ft 6in) tall, you divide your weight (89) by your height squared (1.7 × 1.7 = 2.89). So the calculation is:

$$89 \text{ divided by } 2.89 = 30.79$$

As this is over the 30 mark, you would be considered to be well out of the accepted range for your size and need to take action to reduce the risk that all that excess weight is causing to your health.

Let's take another example. If you're around 52 kilos (which is approximately 8st 2lb) and your height is 1.55 metres (around 5ft 2in), you divide your weight (52) by your height squared (1.55 × 1.55 = 2.4). So, the calculation looks like this:

$$52 \text{ divided by } 2.4 = 21.6$$

This figure means you are well within the acceptable range for your size and have nothing to worry about.

However, it's my belief that you don't need to be a scientist to determine whether you need to lose weight. An honest look in the mirror will quickly reveal the hard truth, as will unsuccessful attempts to get into last year's clothes. There are the comments made by your 'loved' ones, (like 'You're looking a bit fat these days, mum' or 'Are you sure that chair will take your weight?') or even well-meaning friends who try to appease you with 'but everyone puts on weight as they get older'. (Incidentally, they don't and there is no physiological reason that says they have to, either.)

If you don't trust your friends, your family or even your mirror, the 'pinch and pull test' can never fail to be ruthlessly honest. All you do is try to pinch a fold of skin around your waist with your thumb and forefinger. Remember you are pinching the skin, not the muscle. If you can manage to pinch and pull more than an inch of fat, then you may need to lose weight!

Exactly how much you decide to lose is down to you. Some people like to have a specific weight to aim for, others are just as happy if they have an approximation in mind and manage to lose around a stone, say. Ultimately, what you decide to lose is what's right for you. You'll *know* when you feel that you've got down to a weight that suits your mind as well as your body. The aim of this diet isn't to make you obsessed with diets, food and calories or to turn you into a diet bore. What it's designed to do, quite simply, is to help you reduce your weight with the least possible change to your lifestyle and your taste buds.

GOING FOR GOAL

Having some sort of goal is very important; it gives you something to aim for and can be a wonderful motivator. However, it is important to be realistic. No-one is going to reach their goal overnight so you need to pace yourself; don't put yourself under unnecessary pressure, particularly if you have a couple of stones, or more, to lose.

And while it's understandable that you'll want to weigh yourself regularly to see how you're doing, don't do it every day. Allocate one day a week for weighing, preferably at the end of each seven-day stretch, and make sure that you weigh yourself at the same time, with the same amount of clothes on. Perhaps, Monday mornings, before breakfast would be a good time. Check that the scales are on a flat surface as anywhere uneven, such as on a thick carpet, could give you an inaccurate reading.

As you've seen in chapter 2, you can expect to lose up to three pounds a week. If you *haven't* lost between two and three pounds, don't panic. Some people lose weight erratically and you could well find that you, temporarily, have got 'stuck' at what many of us have often refered to as the 'slimmer's plateau'. If this is a problem you've experienced then it may be time to reassess exactly how well you're following the diet. Apparently there is little scientific evidence to suggest that this reassuring plateau really exists and some experts believe that it's more to do with the fact that when we first decide to start a diet we tend to embrace it body and soul, sticking to each ingredient and following every recipe to the letter. However, once we've been on it for some time it's easy to get blasé, and a little over-confident – we reckon we know what 2 oz cereal 'looks' like, so why bother weighing it? Sounds familiar? In short, we get less accurate and less conscientious about our food intake once we've been on a diet for a while and this, say the experts, is likely to be the explanation for us 'sticking' at the same weight. So once again, it's a matter of being ruthlessly honest with yourself – either that or you need to sort yourself out a food diary (see page 37) fast!

And don't forget, many women find that they can put on up to three or four pounds just before a period, which, you'll be pleased to hear, is more down to fluid retention than fat retention. So, if it's just before a period, don't be surprised, or distressed, if your scales show an unplanned upward swing. Remember, you want to come out of this diet feeling as good as you look and ending up a slave to the scales won't achieve anything in the long term.

That said, if reaching your ultimate goal is likely to take a year rather than a month, it's probably useful to build in some extra short-term goals which are accessible but none the less quite an achievement in their own right; trying to sustain anything for months on end can, at times, seem an impossible task. So, for example, if you have a holiday booked in six weeks' time, aim to lose a stone by then. Or dig one of your favourite dresses out from the wardrobe, one that you consigned to the back because you could no longer do it up. Say to yourself that within a month you're going to be able to wear it, look good in it, *and* be comfortable.

The great advantage of the seven-day slim plan diet is that it really does offer a diet to suit most lifestyles and you can mix and match meals and recipes from any of the menu plans to suit *you*. And as each of the diets last only seven days, you've no time to feel bored or fed up because you're eating the same thing day in, day out. Even if you lose half a stone in a month, that's pretty good going, and if you throw in some Thin Day menus (see chapter 13), you could lose even more. Also, seeing the diet in a short seven-day stretch means that the whole diet is geared towards achieving at least some success *every* week. So, even if you may not have lost quite as much as you would have liked, at least you know that every week you will have lost something which will help you on the road to a slimmer you.

And if you don't reach the goal? Well, it's still no reason to get so despondent that you want to give in. Remember, the whole point of this diet is that the weight comes off and stays off. So a week or two's disappointment is a small price to pay for a lifetime of feeling as good as you look. After all, the whole point of the seven-day slim plans is to change how you eat for ever, so losing the odd battle along the way is, at the most, a temporary set-back or inconvenience. After all, what difference does the odd battle make when your aim is to win the war?

WHAT KIND OF SLIMMER ARE YOU?

Admittedly, keeping tabs on exactly how much you eat can be a problem, particularly if you're someone who eats while you're doing something else at the same time. We all find it easy to forget about the nuts that consoled us through the weepy at the local cinema, the cans of cola that accompanied us during the gripping thriller on television or the sweets that were swallowed as we waited for the train, bus, or even the children to come out of school. We've all done it. The trick is to be aware that you've done it and try to keep the urge under control. (One extremely practical way of doing this is by keeping a food diary but you can discover more about this in chapter 4.) Once you've been honest enough to admit to exactly what you eat, the next stage is to recognise the type of dieter you are.

As with other things, when it comes to slimming we all have our own, individual approach. There are those who are thoroughly disciplined about the whole affair and will follow each instruction and every portion to the letter, or to be more precise, gram. Others will find the whole business absolute agony from beginning to end. Of course, the idea of the seven-day slim plan is that no one should suffer and you certainly shouldn't feel penalised. As I said before, the only change to your life should be a regular shedding of pounds. That's all you'll lose. That said, we all have weaknesses and if you identify them *now* you won't have to be faced with them at a later date when you might be feeling a little more vulnerable. After all, in any battle, 'forewarned is forearmed'. So, be honest, what are your weak spots?

For many of us there are often times in the day when we feel like something . . . a little extra. No, we're not necessarily hungry, we just fancy a treat. Eating can, of course, be as much a state of mind as it is a state of appetite and it's important to work out your 'weakest hour' and plan for it. When, exactly, do you turn to food?

◆ DIETING DANGERS

ARE YOU A BORN NIBBLER?

If you are, then the trick is to make sure you have *healthy* nibbles to gnaw on throughout the day. In the next chapter you'll find a treats section which lists foods that you can either eat in vast quantities (should you want to!) or those sorts of treats that are traditionally out of bounds on most diets. Each day you're allowed at least one treat (some days it's two), so just choose those that suit you mood and nibble away! If, on the other hand, your nibbling knows no limits, then I suggest you very quickly turn to 'Beating the eating (urge)' section on page 31; an endless appetite demands some pretty drastic tactics!

DO YOU IMPULSE BUY?

If so, when you go shopping, make sure you go with a list. That way you avoid buying what you don't need, or want. And plan the meals you intend to cook for the seven days, allowing for snacks where appropriate, and then write down the *exact* ingredients you need. Don't be tempted to get just a little 'extra' – if it's there, you'll eat it; it's just human nature. Once you hit the supermarket, pretend you have tunnel vision, sticking to your list with total zeal and utter single-mindedness. Avoid all aisles marked 'crisps; snacks; biscuits; confectionery; cakes' and the like. If you don't have to look them in the eye then you're not tempted. And never shop on an empty stomach; it heightens your interest in food and will increase the likelihood of you buying too much to fill that groaning stomach.

DO MEMBERS OF YOUR FAMILY HAVE A 'SWEET TOOTH'?

This can certainly present problems when you're trying to avoid temptation. If it's another grown-up's taste then at least you can ask them to indulge themselves *outside* the house, or at least not in front of you. Even if they don't want to lose weight themselves, as we've seen, cutting back on sugar and fat won't do them any harm either! If you have children, the problem isn't necessarily so easily resolved. You can try banning chocolate, sweets, cakes and the like from the house but you might find your popularity start to dwindle! Obviously try to cut down on what you buy but if you still feel tempted by either your children's or partner's sweet tooth specials, then try keeping their treats in a rarely used cupboard, preferably in a box. That way you don't have to confront temptation everytime you swing open the cupboard door. Out of sight is out of mouth!

DO THE PROBLEMS START WHEN THE CHILDREN GET HOME?

They're starving and it's all to easy for you to join them when they dive into the plate of sandwiches and piles of steaming, buttery crumpets you've so lovingly prepared. That said, it's worth remembering that your children are still growing. You aren't. Unless it's outwards.

ARE YOU EASILY TEMPTED?

Then get rid of, or hide, all known temptations, particularly, unwanted food. If you don't keep any boxes of cakes and packets of biscuits in the house (all, of course, with expiring sell-by dates so they *have* to be eaten) then you won't be tempted by them. Many people say that one of the greatest problems is half-finished packets, so, if this is a familiar syndrome for you then just make sure all packets containing 'diet breakers' are firmly sealed until absolutely necessary. That way, you're prepared for unexpected guests but you're not tempted yourself. If, once your guests have gone, you have leftover biscuits, cakes or pies, freeze them until you next have visitors, or give them away.

ARE YOU HUNGRY BY MID-MORNING?

If so, you can't be eating enough first thing in the morning. You should always aim to eat breakfast, however little. Start the day hungry and by lunchtime your diet will either be in shreds or will have extremely large holes in it.

DO YOU FIND IT DIFFICULT TO THROW LEFTOVERS AWAY?

If so, get someone else to do it for you. Alternatively, start telling yourself that if you eat like a dustbin you've only got yourself to blame if you look like one.

WHAT'S YOUR POISON?

Work out what foods it is that your find really impossible to resist. For example, if you love everything about freshly baked bread (including eating it) only buy the ready-sliced, pre-wrapped breads which tend to be self-limiting in taste and therefore quantity. And if you love home-made cakes, stop baking them. It really is that simple!

IS LUNCHTIME A PROBLEM?

If you're out at noon, you may find the only food available is the fast food variety. If that's a problem you have then you've got two alternatives: you can either turn to our Fast Food section on page 101 which will show you how to make the wisest choices, or simply plan ahead by taking lunch with you (see chapter 6 for high-taste, low-calorie options). All that you need is a simple cool bag which you then fill with some of your favourite low-calorie foods, be it fruit, dips, sandwiches, salads, yoghurts or whatever else you fancy. (Thermos now have a range of products which keep food, as well as drinks, fresh and at the temperature you want them, so there's really no excuse!)

DO YOU FIND IT HARDEST IN THE EVENING?

Maybe it's when you're all watching TV. As the box of chocolates gets passed round, you wonder, 'Will one really make that much difference?' The answer, of course, is 'Yes'. And, while we're at it, can you really say, hand on heart, that you'll stop at one? In my experience it takes a will of iron, the last thing most of us have at the end of a long, hard day.

BEATING THE EATING (URGE)

Whatever the reasons for your dieting downfalls in the past, there is action you can take to fight that urge. Throughout the book, when relevant, I've listed a variety of slimming strategies to suit the occasion. So, in the chapter on Eating Out (page 82) you'll find some useful tips to ensure that you delight your tastebuds but still watch your weight. And the same goes for the Home Front (page 54) which gives menus, recipes and advice for eating at home, with or without the family.

However, on those occasions when you do feel you're weakening there are various ways of outsmarting those dieting dangers.

DRASTIC TACTICS

- ◆ **Exercise.** Whether it's going up and down the stairs as many times as you can manage, running on the spot or a quick warm-up routine (find out more about exercise in chapter 14) – it doesn't matter what, as long as it takes your mind off food.
- ◆ **Carry a toothbrush and toothpaste with you.** If you feel you're tempted towards a sweet shop, a bakery, in fact wherever you *shouldn't* be, then brush your teeth vigorously for five minutes. It'll take away the urge and leave you with such fresh breath that you won't be able to bear to eat a thing.
- ◆ **Drink a cool glass of sparkling water, slowly.** It'll fill you up.

- When danger really strikes, **suck a slice of lemon**. It's such a sour taste it will take away any desire you may have had for anything else. Alternatively, try drinking cold water with lemon. It'll dull your taste buds *and* it's refreshing.

- If you're really tempted by that chocolate bar you've just found buried at the bottom of your bag, **give yourself ten minutes thinking time**. Spend the ten minutes writing down all the reasons you want to lose weight – be absolutely honest – anything from vanity to health. Then list all the embarrassments caused by your size – how many times have you been ignored in a shop, been made to feel a source of amusement at work or your child's school, felt it almost impossible to buy anything to wear that doesn't resemble a tent or something from a maternity department? . . . got the idea? Now, when the ten minutes have passed, take a good, hard look at that chocolate bar and then honestly ask yourself, is it *really* worth it?

- Appoint a friend as your own **personal slimming supporter**. Then every time you're tempted to eat the unmentionable, dial her number instead. Of course, you need to make sure that this is a *real* friend.

- Whenever you're eating, whether it's part of your diet or not, **try eating slowly**. This means chewing every morsel down to an almost gruel-like substance. The chances are you'll be bored with eating well before you finish the food on your plate.

- Don't forget the tried and tested **picture on the fridge** approach. All you do is dig out the fattest, most ungainly picture of yourself that you can find and stick it on the fridge door. For a sure-fire way of making sure every calorie is *really* a wanted calorie, this never fails! And if you can't bear looking at the photo, or anyone else seeing it for that matter, simply keep it in a drawer and just get it out when danger strikes!

 FRIEND IN NEED?

Friends can be a great support when you start a diet, which is good news to any slimmer. They can also be undermining, unhelpful and downright destructive. 'But it's your favourite chocolate cheesecake', they say plaintively as you try to resist a particularly scrummy dessert after dinner at a 'good' friend's house. 'What about just a tiny slice, surely that's allowed?' And as you detect the scorn slowly creeping into the friend's voice you realise, alas, that all attempts at sticking to the diet are about to dissolve into crumbs, much like the biscuit base on the chocolate cheesecake.

Friends mean well, don't they? Well, actually don't be so sure. Imploring you to eat something you'd clearly rather not when they *know* you've been trying to lose weight for absolutely ages is not necessarily a sign that they have your best interests at heart. So, if you really *don't* want the cheesecake, don't have it. You're really not doing anyone any favours by giving in, except, possibly your friend. But that's probably more to do with the fact that once you've eaten the cheesecake there's no longer any around for her to be tempted by. How else do you think she manages to stay so slim?!

Enlist your friends' help rather than letting the diet become a social battleground. How many times have you heard someone say, 'But you don't really need to lose anything', when you reveal you've just started *another* diet? Or, what about, 'But you're so nice and cuddly – being skinny just wouldn't suit you'. More well-meaning friends, eh? Well, at the end of the day if *you* don't actually *feel* lovely when you're cuddly, that's all that matters. And when all your clothes are tight, you feel you can't move and you don't ever seem to be able to make yourself look nice, being cuddly is hardly compensation for feeling overweight, out of breath, and ungainly.

Wanting to, trying to and ensuring you *do* lose weight is about being disciplined and learning to say 'No'. Unfortunately these are things that women have never been terribly good at. Traditionally, women have always wanted to please and, when a good friend says, 'But I made the cheesecake especially for you because I know it's your favourite', it can seem a lot easier to meekly say, 'Thank you, your cheesecake is good enough to break any diet for', than 'Sorry, but tonight I just couldn't'. However, what you need to remember is that you've bought this diet book for you. You're the one who wants to lose weight and you're the one in control, if you give yourself half the chance.

These days it's considered fair-game to knock diets and it's easy to feel that no-one takes yours seriously. Well, if they don't that's their problem, not yours. As long as you are serious about this diet, that's all that matters. So, ignore the comments, the jokes and the overt offers of diet-breaking 'goodies'. Learn to say 'No' when *you* want to. Remember, this diet is for you and if you don't stick to it the only one that's really going to suffer is you.

You've no doubt heard the saying, 'The spirit is willing but the flesh is weak', but when it comes to dieting it's the other way round. It's the spirit that's often weak because it's so easy to give in to what everyone else wants, and so, in turn, give up on yourself. Your flesh, on the other hand, tends to just get wobbly, rather than weak.

THE ROAD TO A SLIMMER YOU

So now that you've identified all those potential dieting disasters, you're ready to do something about them. Use this book to work out your personal slim plan based on food that suits your mood and choose a diet to suit your lifestyle. And to discover just how easy it really is, read on to chapter 4.

◆ ◆ ◆

4 HOW 7 DAYS TO A SLIMMER YOU WORKS

The whole point of these seven-day slimming plans, above anything else, is to give you choice. *7 Days to a Slimmer You* allows you to eat virtually what you want – whether it's take-away, *haute cuisine*, home cooking or even a take-away spud. And it accepts that there are some weeks when you feel you're eating out virtually every night and others when you feel as if you've been chained to the oven for seven days non-stop.

The following seven diets are all split into seven-day blocks to make them more manageable to use. All you need to do is plan what you're doing and where you'll be seven days in advance and then choose the appropriate diet plan to fit in with your week. And if you end up spending one meal-time somewhere you hadn't planned, it's no problem. Just swap the diet day in question with one that now fits in with what you're doing. By providing complete, week-long diet plans, *Seven Days to a Slimmer You* can be successfully used for whatever your needs happen to be – whether you're looking for a long-term weight loss programme or a quick, seven-day fat blitz.

The whole idea of *Seven Days to a Slimmer You* is that it is a diet to suit you, your lifestyle as well as your tastebuds, and so you'll find that almost all the seven diets can be mixed and matched. All you need to do is to pick the one that fits into your week and then follow it. There are separate chapters on breakfasts and lunches, which give a total of fourteen meal suggestions for each, so you can choose from a variety of foods that are all as high on taste as they are low on calories. All breakfasts listed in chapter 5 and lunches listed in chapter 6 contain roughly the same number of calories, so just choose whatever suits your mood. Lunches are also listed as light meals. Generally most of us *do* have our light meal at lunchtime but if not, just swap the light meal option with the main meal one.

To use the following pages effectively, just decide which diet is most appropriate for you for any given week, or day. If, for example, you're eating out most nights, turn to chapter 9. If you're going to be at home you'll want chapter 7. There's also a week's worth of non-meat meals, plus slimming suggestions, for vegetarians and non-vegetarians alike.

Each chapter gives tips and recipes for the best options, wherever you're eating, and as long as you stick to the breakfasts and light meals given for that diet plan, you'll have more calories to play with for your main meal. If you've overdone it one day, don't panic (or worse, give up!). All you need do is to cut down your calorie intake by opting for some of the Thin Day menu plans, which are given in chapter 13.

Once you start you'll realise it's all very easy as, providing you follow the rules, none of the food you eat should be loaded with unnecessary fats or sugars. You'll see I haven't given calorie counts for all the meals listed. This is for several reasons. One, it's actually hard to be that precise. For example, if both you and I were to make a vegetable *moussaka*, even if we followed exactly the same recipe, the chances of them ending up containing the same number of calories are very slight – our scales are probably different, as are the sizes of the vegetables we would use (have you ever seen two aubergines, or even potatoes, the same size?). Also, people prepare vegetables differently and all this will have a bearing on the ultimate calorie count.

And the second reason I've opted for not giving a blow-by-blow calorie content list is that the whole idea of these seven-day diets is to help you to get to know more about the type of foods you eat – how nutritious they are, as well as how fatty. By bogging you down with specific calories all that you're likely to become is a calorie controlled bore, rather than someone who is well-informed about what they're eating, and why they're eating it.

However, all the food included in the diet *has* been calorie counted for you, and nutritionally balanced, so that at the end of each seven days, you end up feeling as good as you look. All that you have to do is follow the menu plans and get to know the foods you should be eating, and the ones you shouldn't.

Most of the measurements given are imperial. The reason I've opted for this method is because, having grown up before decimalisation caught on, I've never quite got to grips with grams. Also, many foods are still measured out in pounds and ounces – whoever heard of anyone going to their fishmongers' for 1200 grams of cod? And it's the same with fruit: a couple of pounds of apples just doesn't sound the same once it has been through a conversion chart!

That said, there are occasions when I've given metric measurements, for example when that's the weight given by a manufacturer. Examples of this are seen in some of the cook-chill foods available where the weights are often given in metric only and so that's the weight you'll find on the diet.

I hope the weights and measures don't cause too much of a problem for you. To help, I've included a conversion table in the appendix at the end of this book, on page 138, so you'll have an at-a-glance guide, rather than have to turn to a page that's buried in an earlier chapter.

◆ON THE RECORD

If you're someone who finds it hard to keep track of exactly what you eat on any given day, then you're a perfect candidate for keeping a food diary. However, if you're going to do this successfully, you have to be scrupulously honest. That means writing down absolutely everything that passes your lips, and that includes coffees, teas, fizzy drinks . . . the boiled sweet you had because your mouth was dry or the couple of mints to take that awful taste away.

A food diary also helps you identify whether there's a pattern to your weak (or maybe treat!) moments. If it happens to be, say, mid-afternoon then you can start to organise yourself so that you're occupied or equipped with a legitimate snack when your next bout of weakness strikes. 'Forewarned is forearmed' and once you're able to pinpoint exactly when you get a snack attack – and why – you're at least in a position to do something about it.

KEEPING A DIARY

Get hold of an old exercise book, lined, unlined, whatever you fancy. Then put the days of the week at the top of the page and rule lines underneath them, breaking down each day's food intake into meals and treats (if you have any!), as shown on page 38 (or you can

	MONDAY	TUESDAY	WEDNESDAY	THURSDAY	FRIDAY	SATURDAY	SUNDAY
Breakfast							
Lunch							
Treat (Time)							
Dinner							
Treat (Time)							
Extras							

photocopy and use this one). Write down the time you have the treats so that you can see whether there is a reason why you're snacking, apart from wanting to!

It's also a good way to help you organise your meals at home – if you'll be having any – as you can compile your shopping list at the same time. Used properly, it should mean that there's no room for deviations! Some people also find food diaries helpful by using them to record 'befores' and 'afters'. What you do is write down what you *intend* to eat on any particular day and then, on a different piece of paper, write down what you *did* eat. You may well be amazed at the difference!

Keep the book with you at all times so that you have no excuse not to fill in the relevant boxes when appropriate. By keeping it about your person, it also means that you won't forget to write those little extras down, should you have any. By the end of each day, your list should correspond to the food listed for that day's diet – if it doesn't, you know you've cheated!

◆VERALL DIET RULES

- ◆ Whichever diet plan you are following, try to drink plenty of liquids, ideally around eight glasses of water a day.
- ◆ Avoid all fizzy drinks (unless the diet sort) as they are loaded with calories. A couple of colas will take up around one fifth of your daily allowance.
- ◆ Keep alcohol to a minimum. 'Shorts' in particular can notch up as much as half of a day's allowance, and that, remember, is likely to be on top of your three meals a day!
- ◆ Go easy on fruit juices. An average glass of orange juice works out at 60 calories, and that's for a pub measure. Pour it yourself and it's likely to be a lot higher.
- ◆ If there are days when you feel particularly empty or you're simply used to eating larger meals than this diet allows for, then try drinking a glass of water 20 minutes or so before you eat. It should help fill you up and, hopefully, reduce your capacity for overeating, however hungry you feel!
- ◆ You're allowed half a pint of skimmed milk a day. That should amply cover any milk used in cereals, tea or coffee.

- Always used skimmed milk instead of full-cream. If you can't bear the taste, switch to semi-skimmed for a week or two. When you're used to that, moving over to skimmed should be no problem.
- If you like your drinks sweet, use a sweetener or stick to no-calorie diet drinks. Best of all, stick to the drink that has the fewest calories of them all – water.
- Try to limit yourself to half an ounce of low-fat spread on your bread a day. Better still, try bread the Continental way – with no spread.
- Avoid sweets, chocolates, sugary drinks, sugar, fruit and vegetables canned in sugar or syrup, foods with added sugar, cakes, biscuits, pies, prepared puddings, all fried food, fatty meat, full-fat cheese, savoury snacks, such as crisps, nuts, Bombay mix and other titbits.
- Beware of all products bearing a 'low-fat' flash. Just because they're low-fat doesn't mean they're always low-calorie. Most yoghurts are labelled 'low-fat' but an average 120 gram pot still contains about five teaspoons of sugar – no wonder each one notches up 160 calories.
- Start reading the labels whenever you can and most important – **if in doubt, have nowt!**
- The only other ground rule that I feel is worth mentioning concerns vitamins and minerals. Latest research suggests that certain groups of people, slimmers among them, may have a diet that is lacking in vitamins and minerals. Of course if you aim to include the right mix of foods (as outlined in chapter 3), you shouldn't have any problems, but so much depends on factors that you may have no control over (how fresh the food is when you buy it, whether it's been in direct sunlight, how long it's been stored for, how soon it's cooked after preparation, whether it's kept hot, and so on). Consequently, experts now feel it could be useful for some of us to take a daily multi-vitamin tablet, and working on the principle of it won't do harm, and may do good, it could well provide a useful 'insurance' policy if you are worried you're not getting enough nutrients. If in doubt, check with your doctor.

Snacks for slimmers

Many diets mean you're constantly denied anything that carries the slightest suggestion of 'naughtiness', leaving you feeling so deprived that you've given in on the diet rather than give up on your treats. Which is why I've decided to include a treats list in this book. Whichever diet you choose, you're allowed up to two treats a day. It's up to you what you have, and when. All that I ask is that you have no more than you're allowed, and you stick to the amounts given. The best ones to choose are the fruity or veggie ones, although don't forget that all treats are optional so don't feel you have to eat them! The idea is simply that if you are likely to nibble, it makes more sense to build it into the diet rather than make it something that breaks the diet, and it provides a realistic approach to treating yourself!

What you actually decide to have really depends when your moment of weakness strikes. If you're a telly nibbler, you may prefer something long lasting, like a tray of raw vegetables with a low-calorie dip. If you're a mid-morning snacker, a crunchy apple or a couple of crackers could do the trick. What you have, and when, is up to you. However, try to do with the minimum of snacks or treats; that way you end up by eventually teaching your stomach to do without them completely. You should aim for making one of your snacks a piece of fruit – what the other one turns out to be is entirely up to you!

Treats

Each one listed counts as one treat, so choose from:
- 1 mini box of raisins
- 2 rice crackers with a topping of your choice
- 1 rich tea, petit beurre or marie biscuit
- 1 crumpet, scraping of topping of choice
- 1 slice pumpernickel bread
- 2 slices packet french toast, with a topping of your choice from the selection for Breakfast Choice One on page 45
- 3 tea matzos, with a topping of your choice from the selection on page 45
- 2 sponge fingers

- 1 Garibaldi biscuit
- 2 rich tea fingers
- 1 fruit shortie or fruit shortcake biscuit
- 1 ginger snap
- 1 sachet low-fat, reduced-calorie hot drink (e.g. hot chocolate)
- 1 sachet reduced-calorie cuppa soup
- 1 After Eight mint
- 12 Smarties
- 1 slice chocolate orange
- 1 Kit Kat finger
- 2 Rolos
- 5 Polos
- 2 toffees
- 2 boiled sweets
- 7 Maltesers
- 1 chocolate from an assorted box
- 1 diet yoghurt or diet fromage frais
- 1 oz soft ice-cream (2½ oz if it's slimmers' ice-cream!): if you have ice-cream with a cone, I'm afraid that counts as another treat

Fruity treats
- 4 oz grapes
- pink or yellow grapefruit
- apple
- small banana
- bowl of berries (e.g. blackberries, loganberries, raspberries)
- 4 oz cherries
- 2 clementines, satsumas, mandarins or tangerines
- 2 kiwi fruits
- 4 oz plums
- 5 fresh dates
- 2½ oz lychees
- melon, up to 8 oz of any type, except watermelon (stick to 6 oz of this)
- 1 nectarine
- 1 orange (medium-size)
- 1 pear
- 1 peach

- 7 oz pineapple
- 5 oz strawberries

Veggie treats
- As much as you like of raw vegetables, chopped into sticks, to chew on whenever you fancy (this is a great grazing food to keep in the fridge for weak moments!)

But whatever else you're doing, when you're eating try to make a point of following the Calorie Code.

THE CALORIE CODE

- If you're worried you'll overeat, drink a glass of water before you have your meal
- Drink as much as you like, as long as it's low-or virtually no-calorie. Ideally, have water (bottled or tap), diet drinks or herbal teas
- Have as much salad and vegetables as you like, as long as they're 'undressed'. If you can't bear undressed salads, choose low-fat, low-calorie dressings and stick to small amounts. The larger the amount, the more the calories. Alternatively, try a calorie-free dressing, such as lemon or lime juice and black pepper
- Eat slowly
- Chew all your food thoroughly
- Put your knife and fork down between mouthfuls
- Talk a lot – you'll not only be good company, you'll also eat less
- Stop when you've had enough
- Say 'No' to seconds

Well, now you know the ground rules, it's time to get on with your diet . . .

◆ ◆ ◆

5 BREAKFASTS

It used to be said that this was the most important meal of the day. Whether it is or not depends on your personal preference but for me, and I suspect many women, breakfast tends to be somewhat of a rushed affair that falls somewhere between waking up and getting out of the house.

That said, research has revealed that without this first meal of the day, children and office workers find that their concentration wanders easily, drivers have more accidents and, apparently, accountants do not add up quite as efficiently as they would, had they had at least *something* inside them.

But regardless of whether you like big breakfasts, small breakfasts or you 'couldn't care what you eat' type of breakfasts, the following should give you some ideas to suit your schedule as well as your mood!

If you're strictly a porridge person and aren't interested in having anything else first thing in the morning to start the day, that's fine. Just make sure you stick to the quantities given. The same applies to tea and toast. However, if you like eggs, do go easy on them and bear in mind that current recommendations advise that none of use should eat more than four a week, and that includes any you may have for lunch or dinner.

Go easy on muesli – even the no-added-sugar variety is potentially loaded with calories, particularly if it's the type that contains a lot of nuts. Also, extra nuts in your muesli will mean that ounce for ounce, your portion of cereal will seem somewhat meagre, as nuts are so heavy! A small bowlful, incidentally (which is your allowance for muesli) weighs in at around 2 oz (or 50 g).

Taking into account the fact that we tend to have more time on Saturdays and Sundays, I've given you suggestions for four weekend 'specials'. The weekend breakfasts are slightly higher in calories than the weekday ones, mainly because you're likely to have more time to spend over breakfast at the weekend – and that means you're more likely to want to eat more!

Remember, you're allowed half a pint of skimmed milk a day, and that includes the milk you may use for any cereal or porridge, or teas and coffees. If you prefer herbal teas, you'll be pleased to hear that you can drink as many of them as you like. You'll see that a scraping of low-fat spread is allowed with toast, although if you can do without, so much the better. If you prefer crispbreads to bread, two crispbreads are equivalent to roughly one small slice of bread, so swap some of the suggestions around to suit yourself. Some breakfasts allow for fruit juice (choose from orange, apple, grapefruit, tomato or pineapple); a 'small glass' is about the size of a wine glass. Make sure that all fruit juice is unsweetened. Fruit *drink* is not allowed as it's high in sugar so it'll be high in calories too.

◆WEEKDAY BREAKFASTS

BREAKFAST CHOICE ONE

Small glass of fruit juice, if liked ◆ 1 slice of wholemeal bread (or toast) with either scraping of low-fat spread and Marmite or other yeast extract, including Vecon, reduced-calorie jam or reduced-calorie marmalade or scraping of peanut butter, cottage cheese, slivers (30 g, just over 1 oz) reduced-fat, hard cheese e.g. Cheddar ◆ Tea or coffee, milk taken from allowance

BREAKFAST CHOICE TWO

Bowl of porridge (either one using milk from your daily allowance or one that just needs added water). If you need to sweeten it, use artificial sweetener. Plus small handful dried fruit (e.g. raisins) ◆ Tea or coffee, milk taken from allowance

BREAKFAST CHOICE THREE

Poached or boiled egg ◆ 1 slice wholemeal bread, or toast with scraping of low-fat spread ◆ Tea or coffee, milk taken from allowance

BREAKFAST CHOICE FOUR

2 oz high-fibre cereal (e.g. bran flakes) or 2 oz unsweetened muesli or 2 Weetabix (or supermarket own brand) plus milk from allowance, with a little chopped kiwi and banana, if liked ◆ Tea or coffee, milk taken from allowance

BREAKFAST CHOICE FIVE

½ grapefruit ◆ 4 crispbreads, e.g. Ryvita or supermarket own brand, scraping of low-fat spread and/or one of the toppings listed under breakfast one ◆ Tea or coffee, milk taken from allowance

BREAKFAST CHOICE SIX

Small tin of baked beans (reduced-sugar and reduced-salt variety) on 1 slice of wholemeal toast, scraping of low-fat spread, if wanted ◆ Tea or coffee, milk taken from allowance

BREAKFAST CHOICE SEVEN

Small bowl of stewed apples (made with either granulated or liquid sweetener), plus small handful of dried fruit if liked ◆ 1 Weetabix (or supermarket own label), milk taken from allowance ◆ Tea or coffee, milk taken from allowance

BREAKFAST CHOICE EIGHT

Small carton of plain, low-fat yoghurt, mixed with 2 dessertspoons no-added-sugar muesli and ½ sliced banana ◆ Tea or coffee, milk taken from allowance

BREAKFAST CHOICE NINE

Scrambled egg, made with a dash of skimmed milk and seasoning to taste, on 1 slice of wholemeal toast ◆ Tea or coffee, milk taken from allowance

BREAKFAST CHOICE TEN

2 oz no-added-sugar muesli, milk taken from allowance, with a dollop of plain yoghurt ◆ Tea or coffee, milk taken from allowance

◆WEEKEND SPECIALS

Weekend eating should be an occasion, regardless of whether or not you're trying to eat less. So, make sure anything you have is served in the best china or pottery. For 'fruity' foods use a glass dish and spend an extra few minutes on preparation. Then set the table, sit down and savour every mouthful!

SPECIAL BREAKFAST CHOICE ONE

Florida cocktail, made from segments of 1 orange and 1 grapefruit (or use the tinned variety, canned in its own juice) topped with a couple of prunes (either from a tin canned in fruit juice, with no added sugar or cooked with artificial sweetener, to taste) ◆ 1 slice of wholemeal bread

SPECIAL BREAKFAST CHOICE TWO

1 well-grilled, low-fat chipolata sausage, grilled tomato or mushrooms sprinkled with lemon juice, poached egg ◆ 1 small wholemeal roll ◆ Tea or coffee, milk taken from allowance

SPECIAL BREAKFAST CHOICE THREE

Exotic fruit salad made up from 1 lb fresh fruit – choose a mixture of fruit to suit your mood from the following list (some of these will obviously depend on the time of year but when they are available, take advantage!): melon, kiwi, orange, blackberries, gooseberries, papaya, passion fruit, nectarine, tangerine, peach, apricot, banana, plums, grapes, plus a dollop of natural yoghurt or virtually fat-free fromage frais ◆ 2 crispbreads, e.g. Ryvita, or wholemeal roll ◆ Tea or coffee, milk taken from allowance

SPECIAL BREAKFAST CHOICE FOUR

Small glass of unsweetened fruit juice ◆ 4 oz smoked haddock, poached, with grilled tomato, or mushrooms sprinkled with lemon juice ◆ slice of wholemeal toast with a scraping of low-fat spread and/or scraping of one of the toppings listed under breakfast one ◆ Tea or coffee, milk taken from allowance

6 LUNCHES AND LIGHT MEALS

For most of us lunch consists of a quick snack. Ideally it's something that's nutritious, tasty and can keep us going to dinner time. Even if you prefer something more substantial than a sandwich and a cup of tea at midday, the chances are this isn't the time that you eat your main meal. So, whether you prefer something to simply 'plug the hole' that's quick and easy, fast and filling or more of a meal, a selection of midday fillers follows, on page 51.

If you are used to a light snack during the day the chances are you're doing something else at the same time. But when you do eat, wherever you are, it's important to try to sit down and eat properly, rather than taking a mouthful here and there while you're putting the washing on or sitting at a desk working through lunch. Even if you just allow yourself 15 minutes' break, you're at least giving your body, and your mind, time to savour the meal, however modest. If you do eat at the same time as doing something else, it's all too easy to lose track of *what* you're eating, let alone how much.

You may find this is more of a problem if you lunch at home, particularly as you have instant access to as much food as you want! What's important is that you don't kid yourself you're not hungry and therefore try to go without lunch. If you do, all that will happen is that by teatime you'll be starving and much more inclined to eat anything and everything you can get your hands on! So, have a little respect for lunch time.

If you *are* at home, lay yourself a place at the table and *sit down* to eat. Once you've prepared the food, dish out what you're going to eat on to a plate. It there's any over, put it away. Don't put the serving dish on the table and help yourself from that – the temptation to keep helping yourself until the dish is empty might just become too great. And if you are able to eat at home but the problem is that you like the idea of a full plate in front of you, then there's a simple solution – use a smaller plate. That way you get to feel fairly smug because you've eaten a whole plate full of food without feeling guilty about leaving anything!

TIPS AND GROUND RULES

- Remember, all teas and coffees must be made with milk from your half pint daily allowance.
- All bread and/or rolls should be wholemeal.
- As with breakfasts, I've allowed for a scraping of low-fat spread where appropriate but if you can take your bread without spread, so much the better.
- Don't forget that you should be drinking six to eight glasses of calorie-free liquid (ideally water) a day. Apart from helping to fill you up, increasing your liquids is essential to help your body deal with the extra fibre you'll be eating.
- If you're feeling particularly ravenous and worried that you won't be satisfied by any of the lunches below, try drinking a glass of water roughly 20 minutes before you eat. (Researchers have worked out that it takes around this time for your body to start to react) so when you do start to eat your meal your appetite is, at least partially, satisfied.
- Where salad is given as a meal, you can eat as much as you like, as long as you don't add dressing.
- If you can't contemplate a salad without something on top, use one of the range of low-calorie, virtually fat-free dressings (most supermarkets stock a selection), or try a squeeze of lemon or lime juice or one of the new herb or balsamic vinegars now available (all calorie-free).
- Try adding masses of salad to sandwiches, whenever possible. It makes for a much crunchier midday meal and it takes longer to eat. It should also tire out your jaw more quickly than eating a normal sandwich which, hopefully, will mean it won't have much energy left over for anything else!
- If you find a sandwich stuffed to the brim with salad a little too messy for your taste, then serve the salad separately, in a side

dish. It will make you feel you're eating twice as much because you get to have a sandwich *and* a salad!

♦ Avoid avocados. Due to their high fat-content, a whole fruit works out at as many calories as in any of the lunches given below. And that's without dressing!

♦ You can eat as many vegetables as you like (except avocado!) as long as you have them 'neat', that is with no added butter, margarine (saturated, polyunsaturated or otherwise – remember they're still all fat which means, weight for weight, they add up to more calories than the same weight of protein or carbohydrate) or anything else. If you *must* have something, try freshly ground pepper. That way you taste the vegetables, not the butter or margarine. Also give made-up salads like potato, vegetable and coleslaw a miss. They're made with lashings of mayonnaise which makes them high in fat and high in calories.

♦ If you are going to be on the go at lunchtime, take a packed lunch with you. Just choose the foods that are likely to be the easiest to 'pack' from the list on page 53. And to make sure you *don't* miss out on the 'feel good factor', pack a serviette, knife and fork (plastic will do if it's easier) and even a paper plate, if you have one handy. And don't forget a drink. It's a foregone conclusion that any confectionery shop you're near is bound to only stock the non-diet variety of drinks!

♦ If you're 'caught short' one day, in other words, you end up being out at lunchtime when you hadn't intended, before you're tempted to nip into the nearest sweet shop for a little something to 'fill the gap', search out the nearest supermarket or even Boots the chemist. Most now carry a selection of low-calorie sandwiches and some also offer a range of low-calorie salads. If there isn't anything marked specifically 'low-calorie' just look for something as near to 250–300 calories as possible, including some calorie-counted, made-up salads. For more advice on ready-prepared meals see chapter 10.

♦ Diet yoghurts make an excellent 'dessert' for midday. Also look out for slimmers' versions of traditional fromage frais or bio yoghurts – many supermarkets now offer choices under their own label as well as the branded products.

◆ You'll see that most days I've included fruit as part of lunch. A couple of pieces of fruit are allowed each day but if you'd prefer to have your fruit as a snack, in the morning, afternoon or evening, that's fine. Remember, the whole idea of this diet is to find the food that suits *your* mood.

Mixing 'n' matching

All the following meals work out at around the 300 calorie mark, so if you do tend to have your main meal at lunchtime just make one of these options your evening meal instead.

Weekday lunches

As with breakfasts, I've included four 'special', weekend lunches. These have slightly more calories than the weekday suggestions, so be careful when you mix 'n' match – make sure you swap like with like.

Lunch choice one

Open tuna salad sandwich made with 2 small slices of wholemeal bread, tuna (45 g, just under 2 oz) in brine, mixed with enough mayonnaise to bind it (1 tablespoon, maximum) as much salad as you like ◆ Hot or cold drink ◆ Small piece of fruit

Lunch choice two

Poached egg on toast, scraping of low-fat spread ◆ Diet yoghurt or diet fromage frais flavour of your choice ◆ Hot or cold drink ◆ Piece of fruit

Lunch choice three

Egg salad sandwich made with 1 egg, 2 slices of wholemeal bread spread with a scraping of reduced-calorie mayonnaise and filled with masses of crunchy salad ◆ Hot or cold drink ◆ Piece of fruit

LUNCH CHOICE FOUR

Baked potato, with a large spoonful of either cottage cheese or virtually fat-free fromage frais, with chopped chives. ◆ Salad ◆ Hot or cold drink ◆ Piece of fruit

LUNCH CHOICE FIVE

Selection of fresh fruits (variety will depend on seasonal availability) piled on to a bed of low-fat cottage cheese (try the skimmed milk variety – apart from being lower in calories, for some reason it also tends to taste creamier) ◆ 1 roll ◆ Hot or cold drink

LUNCH CHOICE SIX

1 wholemeal pitta. Inside spread thinly with hummous then cram full with shredded cabbage, cucumber, tomatoes and onion to taste or replace hummous by lining pitta with thin slices of smoked turkey ◆ Hot or cold drink ◆ Piece of fruit

LUNCH CHOICE SEVEN

Small tin of baked beans (reduced-sugar and reduced-salt variety) on 1 slice of wholemeal toast ◆ Diet yoghurt or diet fromage frais ◆ Piece of fruit ◆ Hot or cold drink

LUNCH CHOICE EIGHT

1 soft-boiled egg ◆ 1 slice of wholemeal toast, scraping of low-fat spread ◆ Hot or cold drink ◆ Piece of fruit

LUNCH CHOICE NINE

2 oz pilchards in tomato sauce on 2 slices of wholemeal toast ◆ Diet yoghurt or piece of fruit ◆ Hot or cold drink

LUNCH CHOICE TEN

Large bowl of stock-based soup (see recipes on page 61) or choose from a selection of one of the sachets of slimmers' soups (around 50 calories a cup) that are available ◆ 1 soft, wholemeal roll, scraping of low-fat spread if liked ◆ Diet yoghurt ◆ One piece of fruit ◆ Hot or cold drink

Weekend Specials

Special lunch choice one

1 wholemeal bap, split and spread lightly with tomato purée or a smidgin of tomato sauce (reduced-sugar variety if possible), covered sparingly with about 1½ oz grated reduced-fat cheese or low-fat slices of processed cheese, sprinkling of herbs ◆ Piece of fruit ◆ Hot or cold drink

Special lunch choice two

Bowlful of raw vegetables (e.g. a selection of peppers, celery, cucumbers, courgettes) served with a selection of low-calorie dips, either bought from the supermarket or home-made, as follows: 1 oz reduced-calorie mayonnaise mixed with a squeeze of lemon juice and pinch of curry powder, 2 oz low-fat soft cheese, to which you add ½ or 1 crushed garlic clove (depending on your taste) and ½ teaspoon of fresh herbs or 1 oz fromage frais, mixed with 1 crushed garlic clove and 1 teaspoon of tomato purée ◆ ½ wholemeal pitta, sliced ◆ Piece of fruit ◆ Hot or cold drink

Special lunch choice three

Sandwich or large salad made with no more than 2 oz chicken, turkey (skin and all fat removed), or lean beef or ham, cut thinly ◆ Hot or cold drink ◆ Piece of fruit

Special lunch choice four

Smoked fish platter – use around 8 oz smoked fish (trout fillets, mackerel etc.) cut into 1 inch chunks then mixed with salad. Add a handful of halved grapes. Dress with lemon or lime juice ◆ 2 crispbreads ◆ Hot or cold drink

For other light meals, or some substantial midday fillers, see the Fat Days and Thin Days menu plans in chapters 12 and 13.

7 ON THE HOME FRONT

When you're on a diet, eating at home can be a blessing or a curse, depending on your point of view. If you're organised and disciplined, then the chances are you'll have no problem following this diet because you know that the best way to be a successful slimmer is to follow the rules. On the other hand, if you see your home as a trove of temptation rather than a dieter's haven, then you need to make sure that you've got some quick, emergency tactics up your sleeve!

To begin with, particularly if you are used to eating larger amounts, there might be moments of weakness, when the rumbling tummy strikes. However, stomachs do learn to expect less – just think of how tentative you are about eating after an attack of the 'flu or a stomach bug. So think of yourself as the teacher; show your stomach how good it can feel on anything from 1000 to 1200 calories a day and watch it respond by shrinking – the only thing you'll feel is so much better, and slimmer.

Always make a point of sitting down to eat. Being an 'unconscious' eater (someone who's eating without thinking) is a habit, and a habit that needs breaking fast. It's only when you start to become aware of *what* you're eating, and how much, that you are really in a position to make decisions about a 'good' diet. And if you want further food for thought on the subject, all the research on people who are overweight reveals that part of the problem is that we're not aware of what we've eaten on any given day. And let's face it, when you think back, how many times do you remember eating a chocolate bar while you're reading the paper or when you're standing waiting for the bus or train? So, if you don't think when you eat, you're a good candidate for using a food diary, as outlined in chapter 4. It's one foolproof way of really keeping track of your food. And here are some more tips for successful slimming at home:

TIPS AND GROUND RULES

- Reduce the amount you eat by including soups in your diet (the low-fat variety, which generally means stock-based. See the recipes on page 61).
- Use a smaller plate – that way you get the chance to eat a seemingly huge portion (a full, small plate is an awful lot more satisfying than a modestly filled, large one).
- Be generous with spices and herbs in cooking. They contribute infinitely to the taste of a dish yet they don't contain a single calorie. Also, if you prefer different spices and herbs to the ones I've suggested, where appropriate, swap them for whatever is your preference. Remember, the more this diet suits your mood as well as your tastes, the more chance there is that you'll stick to it.
- Dish up your food before you take it to the table. That way you won't be tempted by seconds when you don't really want them.
- Throw away leftovers that you think you may be tempted to eat. If you can't bear the thought of throwing food away, put leftovers in a closed container well out of sight for someone else to eat.
- Enlist the support of your partner and family. If they don't insist on high-fat, high-sugar foods, then you won't be tempted to eat them. And remember, this diet is based on guidelines for healthy eating, an approach that we could *all* benefit from.

MIXING 'N' MATCHING

Each day a specific breakfast or lunch is offered, but if the suggestion is not to your taste, you can refer back to the breakfast or lunch chapters and substitute one of the others that are listed that is more suited to your mood and your taste. Just make sure you're swapping like with like. For example, if you don't like the suggestion for a weekday lunch, you need to be sure that your swap is another week-day lunch, as opposed to one from the Weekend Specials.

All starters and all desserts are roughly the same number of calories, so pick whichever one suits you and your family. You should be aiming for two courses, so choose either a starter or a pudding to go with your main meal. Remember, you can't have both – a starter means no pud! If you're feeling that hungry, then you need to be using some of the recipes from the Fat Days chapter as these meals are high in bulk but low in calories.

If you're a vegetarian, or simply enjoy eating no-meat meals, then you'll find a seven-day vegetarian eating plan in chapter 8, plus some general slimming guidelines for non-meat eaters.

As you'll see, treats are built in to each day's diet but it's up to you when you eat them. Some people prefer teatime treats, others may want to store them up for the evening. Each day's plan indicates how many treats you can have from the treats list which is on page 41. If you're feeling hungry in between meals, I suggest you make one of your treats a piece of fruit, which is more filling than some of the other treats on offer. On the other hand, if you're happy to do without your treats, so much the better – it just means you get to your goal that bit quicker! And remember, stick to the Calorie Code!

THE CALORIE CODE

- A glass of water 20 minutes or so before you sit down to eat will mean that you won't actually feel like eating so much, as drinking can help fill the stomach which in turn reduces the appetite
- Drink as much as you like, as long as it's low- or virtually no-calorie. Ideally have water (bottled or tap), diet drinks or herbal/fruit teas
- Don't forget you should be drinking eight glasses of water a day. Apart from being important because it helps digest the increase in dietary fibre that you'll be eating, it will also give you an increased feeling of fullness, which is particularly helpful if you're used to eating a lot.
- Have as much salad and vegetables as you like, as long as they're 'undressed'. If you really can't go without something on your salad, choose one of the oil-free, or virtually fat-free, dressings. Most are no more than 10 calories a dessertspoon, and you'd never know the difference!
- Chew your food slowly. It's better for your digestion, good for the teeth and means you'll actually get to taste your food ▶

- Put your knife down between mouthfuls
- Stop when you've had enough
- Say 'No' to seconds
- Remember, milk for coffees and teas needs to come out of your daily half pint skimmed milk allowance (it often helps if you measure the half pint out at the beginning of the day and keep it separate from the rest of the family's milk)
- All bread or rolls should be wholemeal, as should pasta. And opt for brown rice rather than white

* Indicates the recipe is given at the end of the chapter. All main course meals serve four people. Choose either a starter or a pud. If you must have both, then you'll have to forego one of your treats.

THE SEVEN-DAY PLAN

DAY ONE

Breakfast
2 oz high-fibre cereal, like bran breakfast cereals or 2 oz unsweet-ened muesli or 2 Weetabix (or supermarket own brand) with either a spoonful of stewed fruit or a little chopped banana, kiwi or orange ◆ Milk taken from allowance ◆ Tea or coffee

Lunch
Egg salad sandwich made with 1 egg, 2 slices of wholemeal bread, spread with a scraping of reduced-calorie mayonnaise and filled with lots of crunchy salad ◆ Hot or cold drink ◆ Piece of fruit or diet yoghurt/fromage frais

Main meal
½ grapefruit, if necessary sweetened with granulated sweetener ◆ Hot Tuna Topping Pasta* served with salad ◆ Baked apple*

Treats
Choose 2 today

Day two

Breakfast
Small glass of fruit juice ◆ 1 slice of wholemeal toast, with either scraping of low-fat spread (optional) and one of the following toppings: a little reduced-sugar jam, reduced-sugar marmalade or thinly spread peanut butter, Marmite (or other yeast extract, including Vecon), cottage cheese, sliver of reduced-fat hard cheese, thinly spread reduced-calorie cream cheese (fruit or herbs variety if liked) ◆ Tea or coffee

Lunch
1 wholemeal pitta, inside spread with a little hummous (about 1 oz) and stuffed full of shredded cabbage or lettuce, cucumber, tomatoes and spring onions ◆ Hot or cold drink ◆ Piece of fruit or diet yoghurt

Main meal
Soup* (choose from Carrot and Coriander*, Tomato*, Onion*, Scotch Broth*, or Courgette*) ◆ Chicken Thyme* served with salad or steamed vegetables of your choice ◆ Rhubarb and Raisins*

Treats
Choose 2 today

Day three

Breakfast
Small glass of fruit juice ◆ Boiled egg, 2 crispbreads, scraping of low-fat spread and topping chosen from list given for breakfast on day two ◆ Tea or coffee

Lunch
Sandwich made from 2 slices of wholemeal bread, with 2 oz (50 g) lean chicken (all skin and fat removed) or lean beef, ham or pork plus lots of crunchy lettuce, cucumber, tomatoes, cress . . . or any other salad stuff you happen to have in the fridge! If liked, spread the bread very thinly with reduced-calorie mayonnaise and black pepper ◆ Hot or cold drink ◆ Small piece of fruit or diet yoghurt

Main meal
Grapefruit Cocktail* ◆ Prawn or Chicken Curry* ◆ 'Cup' of Green
Goodness*

Treats
Choose 2 today

DAY FOUR

Breakfast
2 oz bran cereal or unsweetened muesli or 2 Weetabix (or supermarket own brand) with a little chopped fruit. Milk from allowance ◆
Tea or coffee

Lunch
Wholemeal bap, split in two, spread lightly with tomato purée or a
smidgin of reduced-calorie tomato sauce, topped with about
1½ oz reduced-fat, hard cheese, grated, a sprinkling of herbs and 2
sliced olives and grilled until bubbling ◆ Hot or cold drink ◆ Piece
of fruit or diet yoghurt/fromage frais

Main meal
Soup* (choose from the selection given on pages 61–62) ◆ Tarragon
Trout* served with salad or vegetables and 4 oz rice per person ◆
Jacket Bananas*

Treats
Choose 2 today

DAY FIVE

Breakfast
Small glass of fruit juice ◆ 1 slice of wholemeal toast, scraping of
low-fat spread, topping from list given on day two ◆ Tea or coffee

Lunch
Small tin of reduced-calorie baked beans on toast ◆ Hot or cold
drink ◆ Piece of fruit or diet yoghurt

Main meal
2 slices of melon (up to 6 oz) ◆ Paprika Beef Casserole* served with salad or vegetables, plus 4 oz boiled potatoes per person ◆ Fruit Kebab*

Treats
Choose 2 today

Day six

Breakfast
Small glass of fruit juice ◆ Scrambled egg, made with 1 egg, dash of skimmed milk, seasoning to taste and 1 slice of wholemeal toast ◆ Tea or coffee

Lunch
Prawn sandwich, made with 2 oz prawns, squeeze of lemon, black pepper, and lots of crunchy salad ◆ Hot or cold drink ◆ Piece of fruit or diet yoghurt

Main meal
Soup* (choose from selection given on pages 61–62) ◆ Saucy Fish*, served with salad or vegetables plus baked potatoes (yours to be no more than 6 oz) ◆ Boozy Pineapple*

Treats
Choose 2 today

Day seven

Breakfast
2 oz porridge or bran breakfast or 2 Weetabix (or supermarket own brand), dollop of low-fat natural yoghurt, milk from allowance ◆ Tea or coffee

Lunch
2 oz pilchards in tomato sauce on 2 slices of toast ◆ Hot or cold drink ◆ Piece of fruit or diet yoghurt

Main meal
Soup* (choose from selection listed on pages 61–62) ◆ Meat and
Potato Pie* (see Three-Way Meat Sauce on page 66), served with
2 oz peas per person ◆ Fresh Fruit Salad* ◆ 1 scoop dieters'
dessert (see page 69 for selection available specifically for slimmers)

Treats
Choose 2 today

RECIPES

(All ingredients serve four people unless otherwise stated)

CARROT WITH CORIANDER SOUP

1½ lb carrots, peeled and cut into ½ inch slices
1 onion, sliced
1 potato (if liked), cut into chunks
2½ pints stock
2 teaspoons coriander
seasoning to taste

Put all ingredients, except spices and seasonings, into large
saucepan. Bring to boil, simmer for 30 minutes or so – until carrots
are soft. About 15 minutes before end of cooking time, add coriander
and adjust seasoning. When soup has cooled, liquidise. Then heat
when required and serve.

ONION SOUP

little oil
1 lb onions, sliced
½ oz plain flour
2 pints stock
bay leaf
seasoning to taste

Brush saucepan with a little oil, then cook onions for 5–10 minutes until starting to brown. Add flour and make sure it is mixed well with onions. Cook for a further minute or two, then add stock and seasoning. Bring to boil, then simmer for 20 minutes or so, until the onion is well cooked. Remove bay leaf before serving.

SCOTCH BROTH

2 oz barley, washed
1 lb mixed, winter vegetables (onion, parsnip, turnip, leek, carrot, celery etc.), chopped into bite-sized pieces
2½ pints stock
1 teaspoon mixed herbs
black pepper

Put barley in large saucepan and cover with stock. Simmer for around 1 hour, then add vegetables and seasoning. Simmer for a further 20–30 minutes, until the vegetables are cooked through and are tender, skimming soup when necessary.

COURGETTE SOUP

1½ lb courgettes, washed and sliced
2½ pints stock
1 onion, sliced
¼ teaspoon turmeric
seasoning

Place all ingredients in saucepan, bring to boil. Simmer for 25 minutes, until courgettes are soft. Liquidise.

TOMATO SOUP

2 lb tomatoes, skinned and roughly chopped
2 tablespoons tomato purée
2 pints stock
1 onion, chopped
1 teaspoon mixed herbs, ½ teaspoon oregano, black pepper

Put all ingredients in saucepan, bring to the boil, then simmer for about 20 minutes, until onions and tomatoes are cooked through. Cool, then liquidise.

GRAPEFRUIT COCKTAIL

2 grapefruits, segmented
2 oranges, segmented

Place segments of both fruits in four small glass bowls. Top with a spoonful of orange or apple juice and a sprig of mint. Serve chilled.

CHICKEN THYME

Serves six
1 medium chicken (about 3–3½ lb)
1 onion, sliced
3 carrots, peeled and cut into 2 inch 'sticks'
2 parsnips, peeled and cut into 2 inch 'sticks'
1–2 lb potatoes, cut into quarters if large
½ lemon
2 teaspoons dried thyme
a little paprika
water

Put cleaned chicken in large casserole. Place lemon inside cavity and fill pan to about ¼ inch with water, or water plus stock cube if preferred. Put vegetables around the chicken. Sprinkle thyme on chicken and vegetables, and shake paprika over the chicken breasts and legs. Roast in medium oven (180°C/340°F/Gas 4) for about 1½ hours, until chicken is cooked and juices run clear. Keep basting chicken and turning vegs. so they are evenly cooked, topping up with water if required. If necessary, cover chicken with foil for the last half hour or so of cooking.

TUNA SAUCE AND PASTA

little oil
1 onion, roughly chopped
1 garlic clove, chopped
240 g (about 10 oz) tuna, canned in brine, drained
1 (14 oz) tin plum tomatoes, roughly chopped
1 green or red pepper, deseeded and roughly chopped
1 teaspoon oregano
black pepper

Brush non-stick pan with a little oil. Cook onion and garlic for 5 minutes, stirring all the time. Add chopped pepper and cook for another few minutes. Add tomatoes, with juice, then tuna. Break fish up with a spoon so that it 'flakes' into chunks. Add seasonings, stir well. Bring to boil and simmer for about 20 minutes, stirring occasionally, until sauce is thickened. If sauce gets too thick, thin down with a little water. If you like your sauce hot and spicy, add a dash of tabasco or a pinch of chilli powder. Cook pasta, according to instructions. Drain then top with steaming ladles of sauce. If you're feeding a family with a big appetite, double up on the pasta but remember that extra is for them, not for you! Serve each person with 4 oz pasta.

PAPRIKA BEEF CASSEROLE

little oil
1 lb lean stewing or braising steak, all visible fat removed
2 teaspoons flour
1 onion, sliced
2 carrots, scraped and sliced
2 tablespoons tomato purée
1 pint beef stock
small glass red wine
2 teaspoons paprika
1 teaspoon dried, mixed herbs
4 oz mushrooms (small button ones if possible)
black pepper

Brush non-stick pan with a little oil, then cook onion for 5 minutes, stirring all the time. Remove and then cook meat, quickly to seal, sprinkle on flour and toss meat until evenly coated. Remove from pan. Place meat and vegetables in large casserole. Cover with stock, wine and seasonings. Mix in purée. Cook in slow oven (160°C/325°F/Gas 3) for about 2–2½ hours, until meat is tender. Serve each person with 4 oz rice or around 5 oz boiled potatoes.

TARRAGON TROUT

4 trout, cleaned and gutted
2 limes or lemons

1 teaspoon tarragon
black pepper

Brush ovenproof dish with a little oil, lay trout in dish. Cut lime, or lemon, into slices and divide between trout, placing several slices inside each fish. Sprinkle inside with tarragon and black pepper. Squeeze juice of other lime, or lemon, over fish, then cover dish with foil. Bake in moderate oven (180°C/350°F/Gas 4) for about 25 minutes, until fish is cooked. Serve with 4 oz cooked rice each and salad or vegetables.

PRAWN OR CHICKEN CURRY

1 lb 4 oz chicken, diced into bite-sized pieces, or 16 oz peeled prawns
¾ pint chicken stock
2 onions, sliced
2 cloves garlic, crushed
1 apple, chopped
small handful sultanas
1 green pepper, sliced
1 teaspoon turmeric
1 teaspoon garam masala
1 teaspoon coriander
½ teaspoon cumin
1 teaspoon ginger
a little chilli powder – to taste
1½ tablespoons tomato purée
1 teaspoon cornflour, if you prefer a slightly thicker sauce

Place onions, pepper, spices and stock in large saucepan, bring to boil. Stir well and add chicken, apple and sultanas. Then either cook on hob or in oven (180°C/350°F/Gas 4) for approximately 45 minutes until chicken is cooked through. Thicken sauce with cornflour, if liked, just before serving. Serve with 4 oz rice per person.

PEPPERED FISH

little oil
1½ lb white, filleted fish (thick fish like haddock, halibut, cod or coley
  are best), cut into thick strips

1 onion, chopped
1 red pepper, deseeded and chopped
4 oz mushrooms, sliced
2 ripe tomatoes, skinned and chopped
1 teaspoon dried marjoram
½ teaspoon parsley
juice ½ lemon
black pepper

Fry onion, pepper, mushrooms, tomatoes and marjoram for 5 minutes or so in non-stick pan, until soft. Thinly brush an ovenproof dish with oil. Place fish in dish. Spoon vegetables on top, sprinkle with parsley and squeeze with plenty of fresh lemon juice and plenty of black pepper. Cover and place in hot oven (220°C/425°F/Gas 7) for 30–40 minutes, until fish is cooked. Serve with 4 oz rice or large (6 oz) jacket potato and salad.

THREE-WAY MEAT SAUCE

little oil
1 lb lean mince
2 onions, chopped
1 clove garlic
14 oz (400 g approx.) tin tomatoes, roughly chopped
2 tablespoons tomato purée
4 oz mushrooms, sliced
½ teaspoon oregano
1 teaspoon mixed herbs
black pepper
small wine glass red wine, or ¼ pint meat stock

For Bolognaise sauce
Use 12 oz meat. Brush large non-stick pan with oil. Cook onions for 5 minutes until they become transparent. Add garlic and cook for further 2 minutes. Remove from pan and add mince. Cook until browned all over. If there is any excess fat at this stage, remove it. Return onion and garlic to pan, along with mushrooms. Mix well. Add tin tomatoes, purée, herbs and seasoning. Stir well, bring to boil then simmer for 50 minutes, until meat is cooked. Serve each person with 4 oz cooked pasta.

For chilli

Use ½ lb mince. Add 14 oz tin of red kidney beans, plus chilli powder to taste, about 20 minutes before meat is cooked. Serve with 4 oz cooked rice per person.

For meat and potato pie

Pile cooked meat into casserole, top with 5 oz mashed potato per person. Spread evenly over meat and place in moderate oven for about 20–25 minutes. Serve with 2 oz peas per person.

BAKED APPLES

4 medium-sized cooking apples
few raisins
4 teaspoons reduced-sugar jam
1 teaspoon cinnamon
1 teaspoon mixed spice
2 tablespoons fruit juice

Score the rinsed and cored apples round the middle. Place in baking dish, top each one with a few raisins, a teaspoon of reduced-sugar jam plus ½ teaspoon both cinnamon and mixed spice. Sprinkle with granulated sweetener. Add 2 tablespoons fruit juice and 2 table-spoons water to the dish. Bake in moderate oven (180°C/350°F/Gas 4) for about 40 minutes, until top of apples puff up. Serve yours with spoonful of diet yoghurt – the rest of the family can select their own topping!

CUP OF GREEN GOODNESS

2 crisp, green apples
2 kiwi fruits
2 oz green grapes
1 tablespoon white wine
fresh mint

Core and slice the apples thinly and place in serving bowl. Add the kiwis, peeled, sliced and cut in half, plus the green grapes, halved. Mix gently, add the white wine, if liked, plus some fresh mint. Chill before serving. Serve in individual glass dishes.

Jacket Bananas

Place 4 small bananas, still in skins, on baking sheet or in ovenproof dish. Place in oven (180°C/350°F/Gas 4) for 20 minutes. When cooked, slit open and serve with a spoonful of yoghurt or virtually fat-free fromage frais.

Boozy Pineapple

Cut ½ fresh pineapple into thin slices, then cut into quarters. Lay on flat plate and spinkle with a tablespoon of Cointreau. Chill in fridge before serving.

Rhubarb and Raisins

1–1½ lb rhubarb
1 oz raisins
2 tablespoons low-calorie drink or fruit juice plus ¼ pint water
1 teaspoon cinnamon
sweetener, to taste
grated rind ½ orange

Stew the rhubarb and raisins in the low-calorie drink or fruit juice plus water. Add the cinnamon. Add sweetener to taste plus grated orange rind. Simmer until soft.

Fruit Kebabs

1 pear, cut into chunks
1 banana, cut into 1 inch slices
2 oz seedless grapes, kept whole
½ mango, cut into chunks
peach and apricots (if fresh not available, used tinned variety, canned in own juice) cut into chunks

Brush fruit with lemon juice to stop it discolouring, then thread on to metal skewers, alternating fruits, depending on colour. Sprinkle with a little icing sugar. Grill kebabs for around 5 minutes, turning regularly, until fruit turns golden brown. Serve.

DIETERS' DESSERT

2 small scoops of Wall's *Too Good To Be True* frozen dessert or St Ivel's *Shape* ice-cream or Boots' *Shapers* ice-cream or Simplesse's *Simply Snugburys* Vanilla Dairy Ice or Weight Watchers' ice creams or slimmers' ice cream bombes (have just the one), or sorbets or water ice. (If vegetarian, check labels, as some dieters' desserts contain gelatine.)

Or as an alternative to any of these sweets, you could always have a small bowl of fresh fruit salad, making the most of whatever is in season. Mix in a tablespoon of fruit juice of your choice and chill well before serving.

◆ ◆ ◆

8 THE VEGGIE WAY

You don't have to be a card-carrying member of the Vegetarian Society to read this chapter; it should be useful for anyone interested in cooking, and eating, non-meat meals, whether it's every day or once a month.

Traditionally, vegetarians have always been a healthy lot – not least because their diets were generally low in fat. However, the fast food revolution has meant that vegetarians could now well be consuming as much fat as their carnivorous contemporaries. In fact nowadays it's as easy to have an unhealthy vegetarian diet as it is to have an unhealthy meat-based one.

For example, many vegetarian ingredients are served up in pies and pastries, and a cheese and potato pastie is not necessarily any lower in calories than the Cornish variety! And while it's true that vegetarian food obviously omits animal products, which are often hugely high in saturated fat, many recipes replace such ingredients with dairy products such as cheese and cream – all equally high in fat. So, don't think that the veggie way is necessarily an easy option. At the end of the day, regardless of your dietary preference, the trick is to know enough about the food you're eating (and exactly what goes into it) to be able to make the sort of choices that benefit your health as well as your waistline.

Before you start this seven-day diet, it will help if you're familiar with some of the pitfalls of vegetarian eating, as well as some of the pleasures, so here's some general advice on what to avoid as well as a few tips to help you slim successfully while following the vegetarian plan.

TIPS AND GROUND RULES

- Beware of all the non-meat foods that are high in fat: nuts, avocados, olives, some vegetable pâtés (check labels), many vegetarian sausages, burgers, some frozen meals, as well as all vegetable oils and margarines.
- Many people who cut out meat greatly increase the amount of cheese they eat and hard cheese, in particular, is high in fat and therefore calories. Try increasing other forms of protein instead, such as beans, pulses and cereals.
- When using dairy products, make sure you always opt for the low-fat versions, such as cottage cheese and skimmed milk. (Vegetarian cheeses may be lower in calories but not necessarily so – always check the label.)
- For vegetarians, as a general rule, pasta, potatoes, beans, bread, rice, fruit and vegetables should form the bulk of your diet. These are the foods that fill you up, rather than filling you out . . .
- Look out for *tofu* (a soya bean curd). It's exceedingly low in fat and is versatile enough to be perfect for stir-fries as well as puddings.
- Another vegetable protein product to try, if you haven't already, is *Quorn* a myco-protein that's a distant relative of the mushroom. It is already used in a number of ready-prepared meals but is now also available as a raw ingredient which can be used in a variety of recipes (see Quorn packets for instructions). The advantage of Quorn is that, apart from being low in fat and high in protein, its light, savoury taste allows it readily to absorb the flavours of any of the food that you cook with it.
- Avoid pies, quiches and such like. While the filling itself may not be too bad, the fat in the pastry can turn a dieter's delight into a slimmer's nightmare.
- If you are vegetarian it's important, for women in particular, to make sure there's enough calcium in your diet, so in addition to low-fat dairy products, eat plenty of green vegetables, sesame seeds, wholemeal bread or any type of wheat.
- Ensure you get enough iron by eating plenty of leafy vegetables and unrefined cereals, especially wholemeal bread.

◆ Depending on your overall diet, some vegetarians, and most vegans, may benefit from taking B12 or vitamin D, others may need extra iron. If you're worried that your diet is lacking in some way, talk to your doctor about what would be an appropriate supplement.

MIXING 'N' MATCHING

As with all the plans, you're allowed half a pint of skimmed milk daily (for hot drinks as well as cereal). Meals from each plan can be mixed and matched, so, if you're eating out once but eating at home for the rest of this week, select the appropriate day's meals from the eating out menu (Italian, or whatever you're having) and choose the other six days' meals from this chapter.

I have given a menu for a three course meal but that's only because some people love their puds, while others like an appetiser. However, your aim is to eat only two courses; whether you prefer to have a sweet rather than a starter is entirely up to you. Just be sure to resist having both!

Each day a specific breakfast and lunch is offered. If you don't like my suggestions for any of the breakfasts or lunches in this chapter, simply refer back to chapters 5 and 6 to find something you prefer and then swap the food accordingly but be sure to swap like for like.

I've included yoghurts and fromage frais for some of the days' lunches but do check labels of individual brands as some manufacturers use gelatine as a thickener, whereas others use carob or guar gum. Gelatine is also used in some slimmers' desserts, so once again, check individual labels.

As you'll see, treats are built into each day's diet and it's obviously up to you what you have, and when. If you're feeling hungry between meals, have a piece of fruit, as that's the most filling of the treats on offer. And if you're happy to go without your treats so much the better – remember it just means you get to your goal that bit quicker! And remember to stick to the calorie code!

THE CALORIE CODE

- If you're worried you'll overeat, drink a glass of water before meal-times
- Drink as much as you like – as long as it's low- or virtually no-calorie (remember you should be aiming to drink eight glasses of water a day). Ideally have water (bottled or tap), diet drinks or herbal/fruit teas
- Have as much salad and vegetables as you like – as long as they're 'undressed', or use a little low-fat, low-calorie dressing
- Eat slowly
- Chew all your food thoroughly
- Put your knife and fork down between mouthfuls
- Stop when you've had enough
- Say 'No' to seconds

And remember, you don't have to be vegetarian to enjoy the dishes listed in this chapter. The meals provide all-round nourishment, so you needn't worry whether you're getting the balance right – it's already been done for you!

*Indicates the recipe follows at the end of the chapter.

THE SEVEN-DAY PLAN

DAY ONE

Breakfast
Small glass of fruit juice ◆ 1 slice of wholemeal toast plus either scraping of low fat spread or a little reduced-sugar jam or reduced-sugar marmalade or thinly spread peanut butter or vegetarian yeast extract (e.g. Vecon), cottage cheese or skimmed milk soft cheese

Lunch
1 wholemeal pitta, spread inside with hummous and stuff full of shredded cabbage or lettuce, cucumber, tomatoes and onions ◆ Hot or cold drink ◆ Piece of fruit or diet yoghurt/fromage frais

Main meal
Soup* from selection (see page 61) ◆ Ratatouille Pasta* ◆ Boozy Pineapple* (see page 68)

Treats
Choose 1 from the list on page 41

DAY TWO

Breakfast
2 oz bran breakfast cereal or unsweetened muesli or Weetabix (or supermarket own brand), milk taken from allowance ◆ Tea or coffee

Lunch
Scrambled egg made with 1 egg, dash of milk and seasoning. 1 sliced tomato, plus slice of toast, scraping of low-fat spread ◆ Diet yoghurt/fromage frais ◆ Piece of fruit ◆ Hot or cold drink

Main meal
½ grapefruit (sprinkle on a little artificial sweetener, if liked) ◆ Chickpea Casserole* ◆ Rhubarb and Raisins* (see page 68)

Treats
Choose up to 2 from the list on page 41

DAY THREE

Breakfast
Bowl of porridge (one that uses milk from your allowance or one that only needs water to mix). If it's not sweet enough for your taste, add granulated sweetener. If liked, add a few slices of banana or a little dried fruit ◆ Tea or coffee

Lunch
2 vegetarian sausages, well grilled with small tin of baked beans ◆ Crispbread ◆ Hot or cold drink ◆ Piece of fruit or diet yoghurt/fromage frais

Main meal
Soup from selection* (see page 61) ◆ Yellow and Green Pasta* ◆
Baked Apple* (see page 67)

Treats
Choose up to 2 from the list on page 41

DAY FOUR

Breakfast
1 poached or boiled egg. Slice of wholemeal toast, scraping of low-fat
spread ◆ Tea or coffee

Lunch
Feta salad: crumble just under 2 oz Feta cheese on mixed salad (as
much as you like), plus handful of alfalfa sprouts. Serve with 2 oz
chunk of bread plus scraping of low-fat spread, if liked ◆ Hot or cold
drink ◆ Piece of fruit or diet yoghurt

Dinner
Soup from selection* (see page 61) ◆ Vegetable Curry* ◆ Cup of
Green Goodness* (see page 67)

Treats
Choose up to 2 treats from the list on page 41

DAY FIVE

Breakfast
2 oz cereal (bran based, high-fibre or unsweetened muesli), milk
from allowance ◆ Tea or coffee

Lunch
Large baked potato (about 6 oz), with up to 6 oz cottage cheese and
chives ◆ Hot or cold drink ◆ Piece of fruit or diet yoghurt/fromage
frais

Dinner
Soup from selection* (see page 61) ◆ Spanish Scramble* ◆ Jacket
Banana* (see page 68)

Treats
Choose up to 2 from the list on page 41

DAY SIX

Breakfast
Small glass of fruit juice ◆ Grilled mushrooms and tomatoes on slice
of wholemeal toast, with scraping of low-fat spread ◆ Tea or coffee

Lunch
1 wholemeal bap, split and spread lightly with tomato purée or a
smidgin of reduced-calorie tomato sauce. Top with about 1½ oz vegetarian, low-fat cheese, grated, sprinkling of herbs and 2 sliced olives.
Grill until bubbling hot ◆ Hot or cold drink ◆ Piece of fruit or diet
yoghurt

Main meal
Hot Bean Pot*

Treats
Choose up to 2 from the list on page 41

DAY SEVEN

Breakfast
Small glass of unsweetened orange juice ◆ Fresh wholemeal roll
(look out for those topped with caraway or sesame seeds), or try a
wholemeal muffin, toasted and spread with a thin layer of honey, or
choice of toppings listed on day one ◆ Tea or coffee

Lunch
Cheese and cress sandwich, made with 2 slices of wholemeal bread,
spread with a little low-fat curd or ricotta cheese, chopped watercress, cucumber and alfalfa sprouts ◆ Hot or cold drink ◆ Piece of
fruit or diet yoghurt/fromage frais

Dinner
Grapefruit Cocktail* (see page 63) ◆ Lentil Cottage Pie* ◆ Fruit
Kebabs* (see page 68)

Treats
Choose up to 2 from the list on page 41

RECIPES

VEGGIE CURRY

*2½ lb mixed vegetables – choose selection from: cauliflower (cut into
    florets), potatoes (cut into chunks), onion, runner beans (topped
    and tailed), courgettes (sliced), peas, carrots (sliced)*
6 oz cooked chickpeas (or pulses of your choice)
1 clove garlic, crushed
*1 tablespoon curry powder or: 2 teaspoons ground coriander, 1 tea-
    spoon ground cumin, 1 teaspoon ground ginger, 1 teaspoon garam
    masala, ½ teaspoon chilli powder, ½ teaspoon turmeric*
1 tablespoon tomato purée
14 oz (approx. 400 g) can tomatoes
½ pint vegetable stock
1–2 teaspoons cornflour, if you prefer a thicker sauce

Put all ingredients in a large saucepan, mix well. Bring to the boil,
then simmer until vegetables are cooked and the liquid has reduced
(about 30 minutes). Just before serving, blend in cornflour, if
required. Serve with 4 oz rice per person.

RATATOUILLE PASTA

*1 aubergine, sliced, sprinkled with salt (this removes any bitterness),
    left for 30 minutes, then rinsed in water and patted dry*
little oil
1 onion, roughly chopped
1 clove garlic, crushed
2 peppers (red, green or yellow), deseeded and sliced
about 1 lb courgettes, sliced

14 oz (approx. 400 g) tin tomatoes, roughly chopped
1–2 tablespoons tomato purée
½ teaspoon oregano
½ teaspoon mixed herbs
black pepper

Brush large, non-stick pan with oil. Cook onion and garlic for about 5 minutes, until almost transparent, then add rest of vegetables, including tomatoes. Stir in tomato purée, herbs and black pepper. Bring to boil, cover and simmer, until vegetables are tender (about 30–40 minutes). If sauce gets too thick, thin down with a little water. Serve with 4 oz pasta per person.

CHICKPEA AND AUBERGINE BAKE

8 oz chickpeas, soaked overnight, or 2 x 15 oz tins chickpeas
little oil
2 cloves garlic, peeled and crushed
1 large onion, chopped
1 aubergine, salted, as in ratatouille recipe on page 77, then roughly
    chopped
2 sticks celery, sliced
14 oz (approx. 40 g) can tomatoes
1 tablespoon tomato purée
½ pint vegetable stock
½ teaspoon ground cumin
½ teaspoon coriander
1 teaspoon paprika
black pepper
pinch of chilli, if liked

Cook chickpeas according to instructions. Brush large saucepan with oil and cook onion and garlic for about 5 minutes, until onion is transparent. Add aubergine for another 5 minutes and keep stirring so vegetables don't 'catch'. Add all other ingredients, breaking up tinned tomatoes with spoon. Stir well so spices are evenly mixed with ingredients. Place in medium hot oven (180°C/340°F/Gas 4) for about 1–1½ hours, until vegetables are cooked through, regularly stirring ingredients and checking to see liquid doesn't reduce too

much (add a little water, if necessary). Serve with 4 oz rice, potatoes
or large chunk (about 2 oz) of wholemeal bread.

HOT BEAN POT

12 oz dried beans, soaked overnight (use a mix of haricot, black-eyed,
    kidney, mung, pinto)
1 onion, chopped
2 cloves garlic, crushed
1 lb potatoes, cubed
1 pepper, chopped
½ teaspoon chilli powder (if liked)
¾ pint vegetable stock (more if necessary)
2 teaspoons paprika

Drain beans, place in large saucepan, cover with water and bring to
boil. Boil rapidly for 10 minutes then simmer for about 30 minutes,
drain. Place in saucepan, add rest of ingredients, mix well so spices
are blended, then simmer until tender (about 30 minutes).

SPANISH SCRAMBLE

little oil
1 onion, chopped
1 clove garlic, crushed
6 oz potatoes, sliced and par-boiled
2 tomatoes, roughly chopped
3 oz green vegetable of your choice (broccoli, courgettes, green
    beans, spinach etc.)
1 oz peas
2 oz cooked rice
4 eggs, beaten
2 teaspoons mixed herbs
1 oz reduced-fat, hard cheese, grated
1 oz wholemeal breadcrumbs
salt and pepper

Brush non-stick frying pan with a little oil, add onion and garlic, cook
for 5 minutes, stirring all the time. Add potatoes and green vegetables and cook for further 5 minutes. Remove from heat, add toma-

toes, rice, herbs, seasoning and eggs. Place in a greased casserole dish, sprinkle with the cheese and breadcrumbs. Bake at 180°C/340°F/Gas 4 for 30–35 minutes, until bubbling. Serve with 2 oz crusty bread per person.

Yellow and green pasta

little oil
1 onion, sliced
1 clove garlic, crushed
1 yellow pepper, deseeded and sliced
8 oz broccoli, cut into florets
6 oz peas
4 oz green beans, topped and tailed
4 fl oz vegetable stock
1 teaspoon dried basil
black pepper

Brush large, non-stick pan with oil. Cook onion and garlic over low heat, stirring all the time, until onion is transparent. Add pepper, cook for another 5 minutes, then add rest of vegetables, stock and seasoning. Bring to boil. Simmer for 20 minutes or so, until vegetables are tender. Adjust seasoning. Top with handful of sunflower seeds (try honey-roasted, if you can get them). Serve with 4 oz pasta of your choice.

Lentil cottage pie

8 oz lentils (green or brown)
1 onion
2 cloves garlic
little oil
2 oz mushrooms
4 tomatoes, chopped roughly
1 carrot, sliced thinly
1 teaspoon Worcestershire sauce
1 tablespoon tomato purée
1 teaspoon dried mixed herbs
1 teaspoon oregano
1 lb 4 oz potatoes

Cook lentils according to instructions, drain. Brush large saucepan with little oil, add onions and garlic. Cook until onion becomes transparent. Add all other ingredients, except potatoes, and spoon lentil mixture into ovenproof dish (mash mixture down a little, if you prefer a smoother texture). Meanwhile peel, quarter and boil potatoes until soft. Drain and mash, then place on top of lentils. Place in oven for about 40 minutes at 180°C/350°F/Gas 4. Serve with vegetables or salad of your choice.

For soups and desserts see chapter 7

◆ ◆ ◆

9 EATING OUT

The very idea of eating out can seem a real problem when you're dieting because your food intake is thrown to the mercy of whatever restaurant it is that you happen to be going to. For some, eating out is an occasional treat reserved for weekends or special occasions, for others it's all part of a working day. However, there *are* ways that eating out can be compatible with slimming, as long as you follow some basic rules.

TIPS AND GROUND RULES

◆ Plan ahead. Once you know the restaurant that you're going to, think about some of the foods that are probably going to be available there and decide on the least fatty of the choices, and stick to that decision, come what may. Do not under any circumstances be weakened by comments such as, 'They do the best chocolate cheesecake ever, here' or 'You haven't lived until you've had Mario's carbonara sauce'. (If Mario is that cool a cook, then a request for making a mean pasta sauce that *doesn't* contain lashings of cream and oodles of fat certainly shouldn't cause him to get his spaghetti too much into a twist.)

◆ If you're not sure the restaurant will have something that you'd want to eat, 'phone up beforehand and check. If there's nothing there you want to eat, ask whether they'll do you grilled or baked fish or chicken (no cream sauce or lashings of butter and oil!). If they won't, go somewhere else.

◆ When you're at the restaurant, if you're unsure what something is or how it's cooked, ask! And don't feel embarrassed – the chances are that, if anything, the waiter will be delighted that you're taking such an interest.

◆ If you find the starters more appealing than the main course, order two instead of a starter and a main course.

- If the entrée comes with something you want to avoid (such as chips or roast potatoes) ask for the 'extras' not to be put on the plate. Or, even better, ask if they'll swap them for a salad.

- If you know that you can't resist bread sticks, rolls and other assorted titbits placed strategically under your nose, ask the waiter to remove them from the table. Remember, out of sight is out of mind.

- Don't be embarrassed to ask for no butter to be added to your steamed vegetables or for no olive oil to be poured on to your plate of hummous. It makes no difference to the restaurant. After all, a happy customer is one who will make a return visit.

- Take advantage of the variety of vegetables on offer. They're filling, high in nutrients and low in calories. And even better, you haven't been the one who's had to stand and wash, chop and steam them!

- Avoid gravies and sauces made with cream or/and butter. If you really can't resist them, ask for them to be served separately so you get control over how much you have, then just make sure you add sparingly!

- Avoid buffets – unless you're sure you can resist temptation!

- Avoid anything fried, deep-fried or sautéed (and particularly fatty foods, like goose and duck). Go for roast, grilled or baked fish or meat, as long as they're not in a cream sauce.

- If you feel you have overeaten, don't panic! Simply use more of the meal plans given in the Thin Days chapter for the rest of the week and cut down on all daily treats.

AND A WORD ABOUT DRINK...

Alcohol is an excellent example of empty calories. For your seven calories a gram you get virtually no nutrients whatsoever. And the major problem with liquid calories is that they go down *ever so* easily and before you know it, you've got through half a day's food allowance, and you haven't eaten a thing. Of course there's nothing wrong with a glass of wine occasionally with your meal, particularly if you're treating yourself by going out to eat. However, be sure to stick to one; if you want to make it last, have half a glass of wine and turn it into a 'spritzer' by topping it up with mineral water or soda.

These spritzers are traditionally made with white wine but can be equally refreshing if made with red. Don't be drawn into the 'Just one more!' syndrome, or kid yourself that 'topping up' is not the same as filling up. Also, as a rule, the sweeter the wine, the more calories it contains.

Another sobering thought is that the more you drink, the more you'll stop caring about what you eat. Which is fine, until of course you next weigh yourself. So, say 'No' to top-ups, unless they're of a non-alcoholic, no-calorie nature. That way you'll keep your head *and* your shape.

And beware of low-alcohol, or no-alcohol, lagers and beers. While it's true they won't make you drunk, they tend to have a high sugar-content which means they can contain, at best, as many calories as a fruit juice and, at worst as much as a glass of wine.

MIXING 'N' MATCHING

As with the other seven-day diet plans, you're allowed half a pint of skimmed milk (for hot drinks as well as cereal). Meals from each plan can be mixed and matched. So, if you're eating out twice but eating at home for the rest of this week, select the appropriate day's meals from the Eating Out chapter (Italian, Greek or whatever you're having) and choose the other five days' meals from the On the Home Front chapter. I have offered suggestions for a three course meal but you want to aim to eat only two courses. Whether you prefer to have a sweet rather than a starter is entirely up to you. Just be sure to resist having both – if you can't, then you have to forego one of your daily treats.

All breakfasts and lunches work out roughly the same number of calories in this seven-day diet so, for example, if you'd rather have cereal than bread in the morning, simply choose your preferred breakfast accordingly, making sure you stick to the quantities given. If preferred, breakfasts can be swapped with those in the Breakfasts chapter but lunches here are lower in calories than those given in chapter 6 to allow you more calories to play with when you're out, so stick to the lunches offered within this chapter.

Treats are built into each day's diet, as you'll see, and it's up to you what you have, and when – the choices are on page 41. If you like a glass of wine with your meal, have one less treat for that day. If you're feeling hungry between meals, have a piece of fruit, as that's the most filling of the treats on offer. And if you're happy to go without your treats so much the better – remember it just means you get to your goal that bit quicker! And remember at all times to stick to the calorie code!

THE CALORIE CODE

- If you're worried you'll overeat, drink a glass of water before you leave home
- Drink as much as you like, as long as it's low- or virtually no-calorie. Ideally, have water (bottled or tap), diet drinks or herbal or fruit teas
- Have as much salad and vegetables as you like, as long as they're 'undressed'
- Eat slowly
- Chew all your food thoroughly
- Put your knife and fork down between mouthfuls
- Talk a lot – you'll not only be good company, you'll also eat less
- Stop when you've had enough
- Say 'No' to seconds

THE SEVEN-DAY PLAN

DAY ONE

Breakfast
1 wholemeal roll, with scraping of low-fat spread, Marmite, Vecon, or other yeast extract, reduced-calorie jam/reduced-calorie marmalade or scraping of peanut butter, cottage cheese, sliver of reduced-fat, hard cheese ◆ Tea or coffee, milk taken from allowance

Lunch

Lunch
4 oz pot of cottage cheese (mixed with chives or pineapple if liked), served with 3 crispbreads and small bowlful of mini, baton-sized pieces of raw vegetables ◆ Piece of fruit ◆ Hot or cold drink

Main meal Italian

Starter Melon (it doesn't matter which sort) ◆ soup such as *minestrone* (pass on the Parmesan!) ◆ *stracciatalla* (egg and chicken soup)

Main course Pasta (any sort) with vegetable- or herb-based sauce ◆ grilled fish with salad or a selection of vegetables ◆ fish, chicken or veal cooked in wine or casseroled in wine with tomatoes and garlic

Dessert Fresh fruit salad ◆ sorbet ◆ *zabaglione* (a frothy mix made from egg yolks, sugar and Marsala wine) ◆ Lemon/herbal/fruit tea ◆ filter/expresso coffee

Treats
Choose 2, or 1 if you have a glass of wine with main meal

For some reason pasta seems to have a bad name when it comes to dieting but pasta itself is good news – what piles on the calories are the creamy sauces and the lashings of olive oil. So avoid anything where the word 'cream' appears in the description of the dish or, for that matter, any pastas 'tossed' in olive oil. Anything grilled is fine, although it's always worth asking for the dish not to be laced with butter either before or after it's put under the grill.

Desserts can be hard to resist in an Italian restaurant and if you're not in the mood for fresh fruit, a cool, tangy, refreshing sorbet is relatively low in calories but is still a real treat. And if you want to really 'go Italian' then spoil yourself with the *zabaglione* – it's enough to make you forget that you're still on a diet, and what better way to slim?!

DAY TWO

Breakfast
Small glass of fruit juice ◆ 2 Weetabix (or supermarket own brand), a little chopped fruit if liked, milk from allowance ◆ Tea or coffee

Lunch
Small wholemeal pitta, crammed full of shredded cabbage, cucumber, tomatoes, lettuce, peppers – or whatever other veg. you have available – plus layer of hummous (about 1 oz) spread thinly on one half of the pitta ◆ Piece of fruit or diet yoghurt ◆ Hot or cold drink

Main meal English

Starter Fruit juice ◆ melon or grapefruit ◆ stock-based soup (such as scotch broth, vegetable, but be sure that you avoid anything called 'cream of . . .')

Main course Grilled fish, chicken or liver ◆ stews ◆ hotpots with selection of vegetables (without butter), potatoes or side-salad (no dressing)

Dessert Fresh fruit salad ◆ strawberries ◆ stewed fruit ◆ baked apples ◆ pears in red wine ◆ Summer Pudding ◆ Lemon/herbal/fruit tea ◆ filter/expresso coffee

Treats
Choose 2, or 1 if you have glass of wine with main meal

We've come a long way from the 'good old fry up' and an English menu nowadays is more likely to offer a carvery than pies and mash. Freshly carved meat from a joint can be delicious but it can be fatty. So if you really can't resist the carvery, chicken (skin removed) should be your first choice, followed by beef, then lamb. Be sure to remove all visible fat before you tuck in. Anything grilled is fine, as long there's no added extras (like the odd knob of butter). Stews, casseroles and the like aren't too bad, as long as oil, butter or cream haven't been added. Beware of fatty meat though, as, apart from anything else, it can result in a fatty gravy. Steer clear of any pies with pastry (however much they remind you of how mother used to make them) or 'crusts'.

You also need to give a wide berth to traditional puddings, either savoury, which are made with large dollops of fat, or sweet, which are made with large dollops of fat *and* sugar. And talking of dollops, whatever sweet you opt for, dollops of cream (whipped, double or otherwise) are strictly out of bounds!

DAY THREE

Breakfast
Small glass of fruit juice ◆ 1 slice of wholemeal toast, plus topping chosen from list given on day one ◆ Tea or coffee, milk taken from allowance

Lunch
Boiled or poached egg, 2 crispbreads with scraping of low-fat spread, if liked ◆ Diet yoghurt/fromage frais or small piece of fruit ◆ Hot or cold drink

Main meal GREEK/MEDITERRANEAN

Starter Avgolemono soup (chicken and lemon soup) ◆ small salad with Feta (no dressing) ◆ *tzaziki* (cucumber and yoghurt) ◆ share a plate of hummous. A little pitta bread (a couple of 'fingers')

Main meal Lean meat kebab (chicken or beef) grilled on skewer, served with salad ◆ baked fish – it's usually cooked with lemon, or garlic and herbs ◆ squid, as long as it isn't fried

Dessert Fresh fruit salad ◆ sorbet ◆ ice-cream ◆ Lemon/herbal/fruit tea ◆ filter/expresso coffee – no Turkish or Greek coffee allowed as it's made with spoonfuls of sugar

Treats
Choose 2, or 1 if you have glass of wine with main meal

Greek cooks can use a lot of oil so often it's best to stick to simple foods like kebabs, which are generally grilled over charcoal and have no 'hidden' extras. Mousaka, while very popular, can be fatty and it's worth knowing that it can work out at twice as many calories as an average kebab. Many Greek restaurants' main meals are served with salad, rice *and* potatoes (often roast) so be sure to ask the waiter to at least leave the potatoes off and restrict the rice to a couple of spoonfuls.

Greek desserts can be bad news for a dieter as they're usually packed with nuts and honey. Greek yoghurt may be on offer but with all that cream and fat unfortunately it has to be out of bounds. So, if you *must* have something, make sure it's only fruit or ice-cream!

DAY FOUR

Breakfast
2 oz breakfast cereal (no-sugar-added muesli, bran cereal etc.) plus milk from allowance ♦ Tea or coffee, milk from allowance

Lunch
Choose 1 from the Thin Day light meal choices (see page 117)

Main meal **Chinese**

Starter Stick to soups like Chinese mushroom, vegetable or sweet-corn

Main course Steamed fish (usually offered in ginger, spring onion, garlic etc. or with Chinese vegetables) ◆ stir-fry chicken (often comes with pineapple or stir-fried with vegetables, herbs and spices) ◆ prawn chop suey (which is much lower in fat than the chicken or beef chop suey). Couple of tablespoons boiled rice to share with someone, plus steamed vegetables. China tea

Dessert Lychees ◆ sorbet ♦ Lemon/herbal/Jasmin tea ◆ filter/expresso coffee

Treats
Choose 2, or 1 if you have a glass of wine with main meal

Luckily most Chinese menus give a description of each dish on offer, including the way it's cooked, so at least it's relatively easy to recognise the dishes that you need to avoid. Obviously anything in a batter, or fried, should be given a miss, as should sauces like sweet and sour, but amongst the numerous dishes on offer look out for anything steamed or stir-fried. Rice should *always* be boiled and chicken means fewer calories than meat, whilst fish is even fewer than chicken. Look out for bean curd (*tofu*) dishes which can be extremely low in fat and calories, although if fried, the calorific value of this seemingly innocent dish can zoom up. China tea is optional but apart from helping to bring out the flavours of the meal, it does have the added advantage of taking the edge off your appetite while being calorie-free.

Only say 'Yes' to a dessert if there's fruit which, if not fresh, is at least tinned in juice rather than syrup.

DAY FIVE

Breakfast
Bowl of porridge (if necessary sweeten with granulated sweetener), plus small handful of raisins if liked ◆ Tea or coffee, milk taken from allowance

Lunch
Open sandwich made with 2 slices of pumpernickel bread, a handful of prawns mixed with a little lemon juice, seasoning and maximum of 2 level teaspoons of reduced-calorie mayonnaise ◆ Diet yoghurt/fromage frais or small piece of fruit ◆ Hot or cold drink

Main meal *Indian*

Starter Go without as most starters are high in fat – it'll also mean you'll have more calories to play with for the next course!

Main course Tandoori chicken **OR** chicken tikka **OR** one of the tandoori kebabs. Cucumber raita. Couple of tablespoons of boiled rice

Dessert Mango (make sure it's not tinned in syrup!) **OR** sorbet ◆ Lemon/herbal/fruit tea **OR** filter/expresso coffee

Treats
Choose 2, or 1 if you have a glass of wine with main meal

Indian starters tend to be dishes like deep-fried onion bhajias or meat-or vegetable-filled samosas – both of which are exploding with calories. As far as main meals go, many Indian dishes are cooked in *ghee* (clarified butter), whereas some, like kormas, come in creamy sauces – all out of bounds for dieters. If you feel you *have* to eat something while you're waiting for your main course, ask for a chapati, rather than poppadoms or stuffed naan, although remember that the idea is that you share it with your companion, nibbling ever so delicately as you chat. It is *not* meant to be downed in one go! And always remember that if you do share, then half a portion means half the calories!

DAY SIX

Breakfast
Small glass of fruit juice ◆ 2 oz bran breakfast cereal, milk from allowance ◆ Tea or coffee, milk from allowance

Lunch
Fruit and vegetable platter: chopped fruit consisting of ½ apple, ½ pear, ½ orange and ½ kiwi, plus as much crunchy salad stuff as you have to hand, all roughly chopped. Add a handful of prawns if liked or ½ oz reduced-fat, hard cheese, grated. 1 crispbread if liked ◆ Hot or cold drink

Main meal *Spanish*

Starter Grilled sardines (ask for them to be grilled with lemon juice, no oil) **OR** *gazpacho* (cold soup, made from tomatoes, pepper and garlic) **OR** a choice of fish soup **OR** *caldo verde* (a cabbage and potato soup)

Main course Paella (rice, seafood and vegetables), **OR** casseroled fish, often cooked with herbs, onions, peppers and tomatoes **OR** grilled fresh fish

Dessert Fruit ◆ sorbet ◆ Lemon/herbal/fruit tea ◆ filter/expresso coffee

Treats
Choose 2, or 1 if you have a glass of wine with main meal

Spanish cooking is famous for its use of garlic, tomatoes and onions and you'll find a wonderful selection of fish, all cooked in a variety of tasty ways. However, Spain is also famous for its use of olive oil, which adds oodles of calories in one fell swoop, so you'll need to choose carefully.

Spanish tapas bars are growing in popularity in this country and they're a real treat for nibblers as you can order lots of different dishes which are all served up in small portions. However, be warned that when you add lots of little dishes together the result can be one extremely big dish! Also some of the food on offer is best avoided, however small the portions, for example, the *chorizo* (dried sausage), which is often quite fatty, as well as the deep fried *calamari* (squid) rings. A tapas portion of meatballs in tomato sauce shouldn't cause too much harm on the calorie stakes but go easy on the marinated vegetables as they all tend to be marinated in oil!

Grilled sardines are a wonderful option, either as a starter or a main course, as is salt-baked fish which sometimes comes with garlic and tomatoes and other times potatoes are put into the mix.

For dessert, whatever you do, steer well clear of the *churros* (extremely sweet, sugary doughnuts that have a tradition of being dipped into creamy hot chocolate!). Other sweets tend to be creamy and therefore high in fat, so this is one day when you'll do better to stick to the starter and if you feel you have to follow your meal with anything, make it a black coffee or an inoffensive herbal tea!

DAY SEVEN

Breakfast
Small glass of fruit juice ◆ 1 slice of toast, topping chosen from the list given on day one ◆ Tea or coffee, milk taken from allowance

Lunch
Choose 1 from the Thin Day light meal choices (see page 117)

Main meal French *French*

Starter Consommé ◆ mussels vinaigrette

Main course *Sole Véronique* (fish smothered in grapes) ◆ *moules marinières* (mussels steamed with white wine, onions and garlic) ◆ *bouillabaisse* (a seafood soup that can be served as a main course) ◆ grilled fish or chicken baked in wine, for example *coq au vin*. Fresh vegetables, no butter, or side-salad, no dressing

Dessert Fruit ◆ sorbet ◆ crème caramel

Lemon/herbal/fruit tea ◆ filter/expresso coffee

Treats
Choose 2, or 1 if you have a glass of wine with main meal

The French love their food, they also love their creamy sauces like *béchamel* (made with full-cream milk, butter and flour) and *hollandaise* (egg yolks and butter). In fact, for slimmers the major advantage of *nouvelle cuisine* was that because the dishes tended to be somewhat smaller than we've come to expect, it was still possible to eat French food occasionally and not overeat! This way of eating has lost some of its popularity over the last couple of years but even so it is still possible to go to a French restaurant without constantly worrying about your waistline or your cholesterol level.

Wherever possible go for meat or fish cooked in a simple wine sauce – they're high on taste but low on calories. Cheese can feature quite heavily on French menus, particularly when it's 'hidden' as in chicken or veal for a *cordon bleu* dish (for example, an escalope filled with ham and Gruyère cheese, breadcrumbed and then fried).

When it comes to dessert, many restaurants offer tantalising selections of cheeses but, however much it hurts, cheese can be higher in calories than the creamiest dessert, so ask the waiter not to even let you get sight of the cheeseboard, then you won't have to think about what you're missing. So, when you've got the choice, stick to the sorbets or fruit purées, which are sometimes served with a splattering of fromage frais.

◆ ◆ ◆

10 EASY EATING – THE JOY OF READY-PREPARED MEALS

The busier you are, the harder it can be staying in control of your weight – which is one of the reasons why ready-prepared meals are such a boon. They enable you to keep tabs on what you're eating but with the minimum of fuss. They're also quick and easy to use and their high convenience factor goes some way to explaining how they've become a real dieter's delight.

And nowadays it isn't just the specific slimming products that you need to stick to when you're dieting. With the increased interest in healthy eating, many supermarkets have launched healthier ranges of frozen and cook-chill ready meals. And, as they all contain full nutritional labelling, you can tell, at-a-glance, literally, whether the dish fits into your day's eating plan. For main meals you should be looking for dishes around 300 calories – that way you can have dessert and still have enough calories left over for treats.

Whatever ready meals you buy, do be sure they contain a complete meal (some chilled products only provide the meat, chicken or beans and you have to add the rest). Apart from being not quite so convenient, by the time you've added the 'extras', some of these meals have the danger of ending up not quite so low-calorie, either!

For lunches (or light meals) I've included convenience foods as well as ready-prepared meals. The reason for this is to show, hopefully, that it isn't just foods that bear slimming slogans that are low calorie: two fish fingers, for example, grilled without any added fat, contain fewer calories than a slice of toast with low-fat spread and jam – and that's even when you use the reduced-calorie sort!

MIXING 'N' MATCHING

As with the other menu plans, you can mix and match the food in the sections to suit your mood. And as no-one is suggesting that you live by cook-chill (or frozen) foods alone, just use the eating plan given on the days when you simply don't have the time, or inclination, to do any more than peel open a packet. It's far simpler than slaving away at a hot stove!

All breakfasts and lunches work out at roughly the same number of calories as those in the breakfast and lunches chapter, so if you'd prefer one of the other choices first thing in the morning, or at mid-day, swap them accordingly – just remember to stick to the quantities given.

If you like the idea of keeping ready meals handy – just in case – then it's worth seeing what's available at your local supermarkets. Most of the large chains stock a selection of ready meals, including their own label dishes as well as some of the better known brands such as Findus' *Lean Cuisine*, Birds Eye's *Healthy Options* and the Weight Watchers' range. Also look out for the Boots' range of slimming foods which come under the *Shapers* name. They have a suprisingly large selection of products which includes soups, salads, desserts and ready meals as well as a daily range of Shaper's slimmer sandwiches.

Whatever is the most convenient brand for you, as long as you aim to stick, more or less, to a given number of calories, then you can opt for any one of the ready meals – frozen or cook-chill – available. It really is a matter of choosing the food to suit your mood.

For each ready meal suggestion, I have given a rough guide to the number of calories the meal contains. This is *not* to make you worry about whether you've eaten five calories more than you ought to have done, it's purely to give you an *idea* of what, calorie-wise, some of your meals should be clocking up. That way, if you want to switch my suggestions for some of your own, you'll know the calorie range that you need to stay within. Also recipes for the same dish may differ, depending on the manufacturer (Asda's vegetable chilli, won't be exactly the same as Tesco's) and companies may change some of the dishes in their range slightly which means the names, as well as the calorie counts, may vary.

Desserts are included as part of the main meals. This is especially for those of you who like something a little special every now and again after a meal. And, hopefully, it proves that losing weight *doesn't* mean you have to completely lose your taste for some of the more pleasurable things in life! However, if you're strictly a no-pud person then you can have a slimmers' soup as a starter plus one extra treat, or no starter and two extra treats.

And, working on the principle that this week's slim plan is for you – and your convenience – I've left the choices of breakfasts up to you. That way you get to have whatever you fancy, as long as it's included in at least one of the seven-day diets!

As with other seven-day diets, allow half a pint of skimmed milk for teas, coffees and cereal and try to drink eight glasses of water each day. Treats are again built into your eating plan and it's up to you to choose what you want and when you want them. The list of goodies is on page 41. If you're hungry between meals make all your treats fruity ones, as fruit will fill you up and therefore help slim you down. Of course if you're happy to do without your treats for a couple of days, so much the better – it'll mean that it'll take fewer days to get to a slimmer you! And remember to stick to the calorie code!

THE CALORIE CODE

- If you're worried you'll overeat, drink a glass of water about 20 minutes before you eat
- Drink as much as you like, as long as it's low- or virtually no-calorie. Ideally have water (bottled or tap), diet drinks or herbal/fruit teas
- Have as much salad and vegetables as you like, as long as they're 'undressed' or you use one of the low-fat slimmers' dressings that are available
- Chew all your food thoroughly
- Eat slowly
- Put your knife and fork down between mouthfuls
- Talk a lot – you'll not only be good company, you'll also eat less
- Stop when you've had enough

THE SEVEN-DAY PLAN

DAY ONE

Breakfast
Choose from any of the breakfast suggestions in chapter 5

Light meal
Diet soup (made from a sachet of low-calorie cup soup) ◆ 2 fish fingers, (or vegetable fingers) frozen peas, green beans or mixed vegetables ◆ Diet yoghurt ◆ Piece of fruit ◆ Hot or cold drink

Main meal
Birds Eye's *Healthy Options Steak in Red Wine Platter* or Tesco's *Healthy Eating Cheese, Tomato & Courgette Pasta Bake* (both under 350 calories) ◆ Scoop of diet ice-cream e.g. Wall's *Too Good To Be True* or Weight Watchers' ice cream or sorbet

Treats
You're allowed 2 today

DAY TWO

Breakfast
Choose from suggestions listed in chapter 5

Light meal
Sandwich from supermarket or Boots' chill cabinet — anything up to 300 calories. If you choose one that is 250 calories or less, have a diet yoghurt or extra piece of fruit ◆ If out and about, have diet drink or water, otherwise hot drink made with skimmed milk

Main meal
Tesco's *Healthy Eating Chilli* (vegetarian) or Weight Watchers' *Chicken Supreme Sauce with Vegetables* (both under 250 calories) ◆ 1 portion of slimmers' frozen dessert (select from choice on page 69)

Treats
Have 2 today

DAY THREE

Breakfast
Choose from suggestions listed in chapter 5

Light meal
Tin (410 g) of Weight Watchers' *Tuna Twists* or their 150 g pizzas (both under 300 calories) ◆ Small piece of fruit ◆ Diet yoghurt/ fromage frais ◆ Hot or cold drink

Main meal
Sachet of slimmers' cup soup ◆ Shapers' *Cod and Prawn Bake* or their *Chicken Supreme* (both under 300 calories)

Treats
Have 2 today

DAY FOUR

Breakfast
Choose from suggestions listed in chapter 5

Light meal
2 low-fat beefburgers or vegetable burgers plus 2 oz frozen veget- ables ◆ Diet yoghurt or piece of fruit ◆ Hot or cold drink

Main meal
Asda's *Chilled Cottage Pie* or Birds Eye's *Healthy Options Vegetable Lasagne* (both under 300 calories) ◆ Dieters' dessert, chosen from Weight Watchers' frozen desserts or one scoop of diet ice-cream (see choices on day one or on page 69)

Treats
Have 2 today

DAY FIVE

Breakfast
Choose from suggestions listed in chapter 5

Light meal
Sandwich from supermarket or Boots' chill cabinet – anything up to 300 calories. If you choose one that is 250 calories or less, allow yourself a diet yoghurt or piece of fruit ◆ If out and about, diet drink or water, otherwise hot drink made with skimmed milk ◆

Main meal
Tesco's *Healthy Eating Chicken Supreme* or *Kashmiri Korma* (both under 350 calories) ◆ Scoop of diet ice-cream (see day one)

Treats
Have 2 today

DAY SIX

Breakfast
Choose from suggestions listed in chapter 5

Light meal
Fish steak (e.g. cod) in parsley sauce, plus frozen vegetables, or 2 grilled vegetarian sausages plus frozen vegetables ◆ Diet yoghurt or diet soup ◆ Piece of fruit ◆ Hot or cold drink

Main meal
Weight Watchers' *Beef Stroganoff* or *Vegetable Mousaka* (both under 300 calories) ◆ One of Weight Watchers' or Shapers' ice-cream *Bombes*

Treats
Have 2 today

Day seven

Breakfast
Choose from suggestions in chapter 5

Light meal
2 vegetable grills or fish cakes plus 2 oz baked or kidney beans or low-calorie, ready-prepared salad (anything up to 160 calories for a pot), plus pack of slimmers' pâté (Shapers' have *Garlic, Peppercorn* and *Ardennes* varieties) – anything up to 140 calories ◆ Hot or cold drink

Main meal
Lean Cuisine Prawn Curry, Beef Lasagne or *Vegetable Gratin* (all under 300 calories) ◆ ½ large tin (a large tin is usually around 425 g or 17 oz) reduced-calorie rice pudding, plus a teaspoon of reduced-calorie jam, if liked

Treats
You can have 2 today

◆ ◆ ◆

11 FAST FOOD

Take-aways and fast food can be terrific news if you're in a hurry – they're fast to find (hasn't almost every town got at least *one* fast food chain?), fast to get, fast to eat and, unfortunately, can be a fast way to get fat. However, if you choose wisely then it is possible to take away even when you're trying to slim.

Whichever way you look at it, fast food tends to be high in saturated fat which means it can't avoid being high in calories too, so you'll need to be strong on willpower, otherwise you could easily be tempted off the slimming straight and narrow. It's also worth remembering that any dish with 'whopper', 'extra large', or 'deluxe' as part of its name means whopper, extra large and deluxe calories too – so steer clear! Also if you're ordering a drink with your fast food fare, make sure it's the diet sort – water, or tea or coffee without milk. Fast food chains are unlikely to have skimmed milk but what they *do* often have on offer is a non-dairy creamer which is bad news, as it's high in saturated fat.

The following menu plan allows you to balance the rest of the day's food intake so any potential fast food damage can be kept to a minimum. When it comes to totting up exactly how many calories are in each dish, it's worth noting that cooking methods, and even recipes, will vary from place to place so this particular seven-day diet plan is designed to give you enough information to enable you to go for the lowest calorie options available.

As working out how many calories specific fast foods contains is such an inexact science, the rest of the meals for the day have been balanced to compensate for any unplanned extra calories – hence the increase in Thin Day menus – which contain lower calorie meals and snacks than in the other slim plans. However, if you follow the suggestions given you'll still get to have three meals a day *and* eat out and still lose weight!

Mixing 'n' matching

Each day you're allowed half a pint of skimmed milk (for use in teas, coffees and with cereal). As with the other menu plans, the days' menus can be mixed and matched. If you only have a take-away one day, select that day's menus around the take-away of your choice; if you opt for your fast food meal at lunchtime, simply have the lunch meal for dinner.

If you prefer some of the breakfast options given in the breakfasts' section (chapter 5) to the ones suggested here, simply swap the breakfasts accordingly, making sure you stick to the quantities given. Lunches on this plan are slightly lower in calories than those given in the lunch chapter so only swap midday meals within the options given for the following seven days. As with the other diet plans, you're allowed treats each day, although it's up to you what you have and when (see the full list of choices on page 41). However, they're far from obligatory and if you can do without them, so much the better! And remember to stick to the calorie code!

The calorie code

- If you're worried you'll overeat, drink a glass of water before you leave home
- Drink as much as you like – as long as it's low- or virtually no-calorie. Ideally, have water (bottled or tap), diet drinks or herbal or fruit teas
- Have as much salad and vegetables as you like, as long as they're 'undressed'
- Eat slowly
- Chew all your food thoroughly
- Talk a lot – you'll not only be good company, you'll also eat less
- Stop when you've had enough
- Say 'No' to seconds

THE SEVEN-DAY PLAN

DAY ONE

Breakfast
Small glass of fruit juice ♦ 1 slice of wholemeal toast, either scraping of low-fat spread with Marmite, Vecon, or supermarket own brand yeast extract, reduced-sugar jam or reduced-sugar marmalade; or scraping of peanut butter, cottage cheese, sliver of reduced-fat cheese ♦ Tea or coffee, milk taken from allowance

Lunch
4 oz cottage cheese, mixed with chopped apple and orange (fruit can be eaten separately if preferred) ♦ 2 crispbreads, scraping of low-fat spread, if liked ♦ Hot or cold drink

Main meal **Pizza**
Choose one small, thin crust (as opposed to deep pan) pizza with topping of your choice (see below) ♦ vegetarian option ♦ small pizza slice. Salad, no dressing ♦ Diet drink

Treats
Choose 2 from list on page 41

Pizzas are traditionally high in calories – mainly because of all that cheese. However, nowadays the good news is that most pizza places let you create your own recipe, which means you get to have *exactly* what you want. So, you can specify *no* (or at least, *very little*) cheese, while opting for extras like peppers, mushrooms, prawns, sweetcorn, tuna – the list goes on. Alternatively, if they have a non-cheese pizza, go for that.

If the choice is more limited, have the pizza of your choice but share it rather than having a whole one to yourself. Or, if the pizza place categorically won't reduce the amount of cheese they use, try scraping some off. There's no rule that says you *have* to eat everything in front of you!

If you're going out for a pizza, take advantage of the salad bar. Many chain restaurants now offer quite a decent choice that's a far cry from the wrinkled tomatoes, dried out cucumber and limp, brown-edged lettuce that used to be available.

DAY TWO

Breakfast
1 ½ oz – 2 oz unsweetened muesli, or 2 Weetabix (or supermarket own brand), with a little chopped up fruit plus milk from allowance ◆ Tea or coffee

Lunch
1 boiled egg, plus 1 slice of wholemeal toast, scraping of low-fat spread ◆ Piece of fruit ◆ Hot or cold drink

Main meal **Burgers**
Choose plain, 2 oz burger plus half share of a portion of chips, or 2 oz cheeseburger. If you're at a McDonalds, you also have the choice of 9 *Chicken McNuggets* (or 6 with chips – if you'll limit yourself to sharing a portion!) ◆ a *Bacon and Egg McMuffin* (if it's available) ◆ *Fillet O Fish* ◆ *Quarter Pounder* with a McDonald's salad. If you can't resist chips and do order a portion to share with your friends, remember to eat each and every one *slowly* ◆ Tea, coffee, water or ask for a diet drink

Treats
Choose 2 treats today

DAY THREE

Breakfast
Scrambled egg, dash of skimmed milk, seasoning to taste, or boiled egg, plus 1 slice of wholemeal toast, scraping of low-fat spread ◆ Tea or coffee

Lunch
Tuna salad made with 2 slices of wholemeal bread, maximum of 45 g

(just under 2 oz) tuna in brine (drained), mixed with lots of crunchy salad. Add black pepper and a drizzle of oil-free dressing if liked. Plus wholemeal roll, scraping of low-fat spread ◆ Hot or cold drink ◆ Piece of fruit or diet yoghurt/fromage frais

Main meal *Baked potato*
Choose baked potato with one of following: sweetcorn, baked beans, Mexican beans, tuna (although check it's not smothered in mayonnaise), prawns, curry, green salad (if on offer) and, of course, cottage cheese ◆ Diet drink or water

Treats
You're allowed 2 today

A baked potato offers terrific value nutritionally as it's packed full of vitamins, minerals and fibre and is low-fat, provided you don't add fatty fillings. So avoid hard cheese and mayonnaise and always say 'No' to butter or garlic butter!

DAY FOUR

Breakfast
Small glass of fruit juice ◆ 2 oz bran breakfast cereal, milk taken from allowance ◆ Tea or coffee

Lunch
Prawn sandwich made with 2 slices of wholemeal bread, a small amount of reduced-calorie mayonnaise mixed into a handful of prawns (about 1 oz) with black pepper and a squeeze of lemon juice. As much salad as you like ◆ Piece of fruit or diet yoghurt/fromage frais ◆ Hot or cold drink

Main meal **Fried chicken**
Choose 2 pieces of fried chicken ◆**OR** 1 piece of chicken and a baked potato (no butter) ◆ Diet drink or water

Treats
You're allowed 1 today

Deep-fried chicken is never exactly the dieter's friend but by limiting yourself to no more than 2 pieces of chicken – and passing on the chips and coleslaw – you've got yourself a perfectly acceptable main meal. Some fried chicken chains offer baked potatoes as an alternative to chips, so always ask.

Day five

Breakfast
½ grapefruit, 1 slice of wholemeal toast with topping (choose from list given in day one) ◆ Tea or coffee, milk taken from allowance

Lunch
1 boiled egg, 2 crispbreads, scraping of low-fat spread, slivers of low-fat cheese (about 1 oz) ◆ Piece of fruit ◆ Hot or cold drink

Main meal *Fish and chips*
Choose grilled fish, if available ◆ small fillet of fried, plus shared portion of thick-cut chips ◆ Diet drink or water

Treats
You're allowed 1 today (2 if the fish is grilled)

Fish and chips can be one of the highest calorie fast foods there is, due to all that deep-frying. Many 'chippie's' are starting to fry fish in vegetable oil which, while better for your health, is still bad news for your waistline. Some shops are now offering grilled fish so before you put in your order, check whether it's available. If not, take off some, if not all, of the batter – that way you get all the taste of fresh fish but none of the fat! Avoid those squeezy bottles full of tartare and tomato sauce – one over-enthusiastic squeeze can end up covering half your plate – and ask for a quarter of a lemon instead. As for chips, even a small portion can work out at around 250 calories, and the thinner the chips, the more the calories due to the larger surface area there is to absorb the fat. So, if you really can't pass on the chips, share your portion with a friend, and eat yours slowly . . .

DAY SIX

Breakfast
Bowl of porridge (either one that is made up with water or use milk from allowance) with granulated sweetener, and small handful of dried fruit (e.g. raisins) if liked ◆ Tea or coffee, milk from allowance

Lunch
Banana sandwich made with 2 slices of wholemeal bread, scraping of low-fat spread and 1 small, mashed banana (or ½ large one) ◆ Diet yoghurt or diet fromage frais ◆ Hot or cold drink

Main meal Kebab
Choose kebab in pitta bread with salad
Diet drink or water

Treats
You're allowed 2 today

With kebabs it's often hard to tell how many calories you're letting yourself in for as so much depends on how fatty the meat is. It can be easier to see how much fat is on *shish* kebabs (cubed beef which is cooked on skewers) because it's immediately visible but with *doner* kebabs (where the meat is sliced off a spit while you wait) it can be a different matter. Sometimes chicken kebabs are on offer, which is your best bet, but if not, whether you opt for doner or shish, ask them to stuff the pitta with plenty of salad and if you spot any pieces of fat lurking under the lettuce, remove them fast!

DAY SEVEN

Here I've given the main meal suggestions at midday because if you do eat at your 'local', it's more likely to be at lunchtime.

Breakfast
Florida cocktail, made with segments of 1 orange and 1 grapefruit, or use the tinned variety canned in natural juice. Plus 1 wholemeal roll, plus topping chosen from list given under day one ◆ Tea or coffee, milk taken from allowance

Main meal PUB GRUB

Choose jacket potato, salad ◆ low-fat sandwich (ask for no butter), filled with lean beef, ham, chicken, turkey or prawns ◆ Drink mineral water, diet drink or one *spritzer* (half wine, half soda or mineral water)

Some pubs are really getting into the healthy swing of things by offering tantalising selections of salads, as well as the traditional ham, prawn and chicken variety (remember to remove any skin and fat). High-fibre, low-fat snacks are also increasingly available – anything from jacket potato to vegetarian mixed bean casserole. At all costs avoid anything with pastry (from quiches to sausage rolls) as the fat content is likely to send any self-respecting dieter into slimmers' shock! A ploughman's lunch may look harmless but as most pubs usually serve it with a huge chunk of cheese (not to mention the pats of butter), it's best to avoid it altogether. If you decide on a sandwich, ask for one without butter and if you're having a salad don't forget – no dressing!

However, if your local is the sort that thinks greasy sausages, sausage rolls and packets of crisps is what's meant by customer choice, then I suggest you either eat before you get there – or better still, find another local!

Light meal

Choose from one of Thin Day lunch choices (see page 117)

Treats

You're allowed 3 treats today, (2 if you have a drink with your meal)

◆ ◆ ◆

12 FAT DAYS

We all get them. There are some days when you're running around so much that you're quite happy to settle for something light, while other days you could quite easily graze through whatever food is put in front of you. It's what I call the Fat Day, Thin Day Syndrome and of course, Fat Days are the most dangerous ones for a slimmer – they're those occasions when it's as if your appetite knows no limits!

However, if in the middle of your diet you are struck by a day like this just turn to one of the Fat Day menu plans.

The following diet is devised to fill you up and slim you down – all at the same time! The meals are high in fibre and complex carbohydrates as well as being low in fat and sugar, so it should mean no hunger pains. You'll also discover that you have little, if any, room left to graze, even if you wanted to!

TIPS AND GROUND RULES

- ◆ For Fat Day appetites that really can't be satisfied, remember to drink your eight glasses of water during the day. Apart from filling you up, the extra fluid is important to help digest the extra fibre that you'll be eating. And a glass 20 minutes or so before you sit down to eat should mean that you won't be able to overeat, as drinking fills up the stomach which, in turn, reduces the appetite.
- ◆ One of the tricks to help beat that Fat Day feeling is to eat a main meal in the middle of the day. That way you're less inclined to nibble assorted 'naughties'!
- ◆ It also helps if all your treats are fruit or vegetable (raw) ones as they keep your mouth busy at the same time as filling your stomach. Have a selection of raw vegetables, washed and sliced, readily available for when hunger, greed or grazing strikes!

- If you find that it's the cold that drives you towards the fridge, make one of your treats a cup of steaming, low-calorie soup. Either opt for supermarket sachets or make sure you've got one of the home-made soups (see page 61) made up so all you need do is heat it through – and consume.

- If you've really got a bad attack of the 'eats', pour yourself out a cool glass of water, sit down at the table and drink it slowly. Then go and find something to do for the 20 minutes or so that it'll take you to feel full. Hopefully, by the time the 20 minutes are up, you will have completely forgotten about food. If not, then I suggest you quickly turn to Beating The Eating Urge tips on page 31, for some emergency tactics on exactly how to divert your appetite.

- Remember, milk for coffees, teas and cereals needs to come out of your daily half pint skimmed milk allowance. Measure the amount out at the beginning of the day and keep it separate from the rest of the family's milk.

- All bread, or rolls, should be wholemeal, as should pasta. And opt for brown rice rather than white.

MIXING 'N' MATCHING

Each day a specific breakfast or lunch is offered but if the suggestion is not to your liking, you can refer back to the breakfast or lunch chapters and substitute one more suited to your mood and your taste. However, it's worth mentioning that the lunches given here are specifically geared towards the days when you want to eat more than usual, so if possible stick to one of the lunches in this chapter.

I've given choices for starters and desserts for your main meal but, as with the other seven-day diets, you should have either one or the other, not both. If you want, you can swap one of the Fat Day dishes for one of the home cooking or vegetarian main meals (if appropriate).

It may be that you want to follow the suggestions given here for a whole week, if so you may find that after the seven days you haven't lost as much weight as you will have done on the other diets. Don't worry – it's because your calorie intake is slightly higher on this plan, due to the increase in what you're eating. However, if you stick to the plan, there's no reason why you still shouldn't lose up to a couple of pounds at the end of the week. And if you can cope, remind yourself that all treats are optional; cut them out and you cut back the time it takes to become a slimmer you. And remember to stick to the Calorie Code!

* Indicates the recipe is given at the end of this chapter.

THE CALORIE CODE

- Drink as much as you like, as long as it's low- or virtually no-calorie. Ideally, have water (bottled or tap), diet drinks or herbal/fruit teas
- Have as much salad and vegetables as you like, as long as they're 'undressed' or you use low-fat, low-calorie dressings. Even then, limit yourself to a modest amount as the more you have, the more calories you consume. Alternatively 'dress' the calorie-free way – with black pepper and a squeeze of lemon juice
- Eat slowly
- Chew all your food thoroughly
- Put your knife and fork down between mouthfuls
- Stop when you've had enough

THE SEVEN-DAY PLAN

FAT DAY ONE

Breakfast
Large bowl of porridge (made with milk from allowance or water) if not sweet enough, sprinkled with a little granulated sweetener, plus a small handful of dried fruit (e.g. raisins) or some chopped banana ◆ Tea or coffee

Lunch
Sachet low-calorie soup ◆ Chicken joint, no skin, as much salad as you can eat ◆ 4 bread triangles, made from 1 slice of bread, with a

scraping of low-fat spread ◆ Hot or cold drink ◆ Piece of fruit or diet yoghurt

Dinner
Stock-based soup chosen from selection given on page 61 ◆ Large baked potato with ratatouille* filling (use 2 rounded tablespoons from ratatouille recipe, on page 77), topped with 1½ oz reduced-fat, hard cheese, grated ◆ Diet yoghurt or diet fromage frais

Treats
2 allowed today

FAT DAY TWO

Breakfast
2 oz bran breakfast cereal, unsweetened muesli or 2 Weetabix (or supermarket own brand) with a little chopped fruit ◆ Tea or coffee

Lunch
Bowl of Bean Soup*, plus large chunk of wholemeal bread, scraping of low-fat spread, if liked

Main meal
Curry* – vegetable, chicken or prawn (see recipes on pages 77 and 65) ◆ Boozy Pineapple* (page 68)

Treats
2 allowed today

FAT DAY THREE

Breakfast
Small glass of fruit juice ◆ 1 slice of wholemeal toast with scraping of low-fat spread, Marmite (or other yeast extract), reduced-calorie jam or reduced-calorie marmalade or scraping of peanut butter, cottage cheese, sliver of reduced-fat, hard cheese ◆ Tea or coffee, milk taken from allowance

Lunch
Tuna Baguette* ◆ Hot or cold drink

Main meal
Soup, chosen from selection on page 61 ◆ Paprika Beef Casserole*
(see page 64) ◆ Rhubarb and Raisins* (see page 68)

Treats
2 allowed today

FAT DAY FOUR

Breakfast
Large bowl of porridge (made with milk from allowance or water) add
granulated sweetener if necessary, plus a little chopped fruit ◆ Tea
or coffee

Lunch
Double decker sandwich made with 3 slices of wholemeal bread. On
1 slice place 1 oz smoked turkey, plus masses of crunchy salad
(scraping of reduced-calorie mayonnaise, if wanted), place another
slice on top and cover with 1 oz either pastrami or lean ham, pile on
more salad and reduced-calorie mayonnaise, if wanted) then top with
last slice of bread. Cut into triangles and proceed to eat, keeping
plenty of serviettes handy!

Main meal
Soup chosen from selection given on page 61 ◆ Large bowl of Chilli*
(see Three-Way Meat recipe on page 66) ◆ Fruit of choice

Treats
2 allowed today

FAT DAY FIVE

Breakfast
1 slice of wholemeal toast, scaping of low-fat spread, 1 boiled egg ◆
Tea or coffee

Lunch
Seafood Special* ◆ Diet fromage frais or diet yoghurt ◆ Piece of fruit ◆ Hot or cold drink

Main meal
Soup chosen from selection given on page 61 ◆ Large tin (400 g, 1 lb) vegetable or tuna ravioli, served with salad or selection of vegetables ◆ 2 scoops of diet ice-cream (see page 69 for selection)

Treats
2 allowed today

FAT DAY SIX

Breakfast
Bowl of porridge (made with either milk from allowance or water) plus half a banana or small handful of dried fruit. Use granulated sweetener if necessary. ◆ Tea or coffee

Lunch
Large baked potato with 4 rounded tablespoons of Three-Way Meat Sauce* (see recipe on page 66) ◆ Piece of fruit or diet yoghurt ◆ Hot or cold drink

Main meal
½ grapefruit ◆ Tuna Sauce and Pasta* (see recipe on page 63) ◆ If wanted, fruit-based dessert from choice given on pages 67–68

Treats
2 allowed today

FAT DAY SEVEN

Breakfast
Bowl of porridge (as day six) or 2 oz breakfast cereal (as day two) ◆ Tea or coffee

Lunch
Sachet of low-calorie soup ◆ Bit of Everything Salad* ◆ Piece of
fruit or diet yoghurt ◆ Hot or cold drink

Main meal
Soup chosen from selection given on page 61 ◆ Hot Bean Pot* (see
recipe on page 79) ◆ Fruit kebab* (see recipe on page 68)

Treats
2 allowed today

RECIPES

THICK BEAN SOUP

8 oz dried beans, soaked according to instructions, and drained (use
black-eyed beans, kidney beans or aduki beans)
1 onion, chopped
2 sticks celery, sliced
2 carrots, sliced
1 tablespoon tomato purée
1 teaspoon mixed herbs
black pepper
2½ pints vegetable stock

Put beans and stock into large saucepan, bring to boil. Boil for 10
minutes then add all other ingredients. Stir well and simmer for
approximately 50 minutes, until beans are cooked through. Adust
seasoning. If preferred, try liquidising either all, or two thirds of the
soup to make a rich and filling meal. Serve with thick slice of wholemeal bread.

SEAFOOD SPECIAL

6 oz peeled prawns
4 oz wholemeal pasta, cooked
2 spring onions, sliced thinly
2 sticks celery, sliced

2 courgettes, sliced
1 head of fennel, sliced
lettuce
lemon juice or splash of oil-free or low-fat dressing
black pepper

Mix cooked prawns, pasta and spring onions with splash of dressing. Pile mixture on to bed of lettuce, fennel and courgettes (or anything else you happen to have lying around!). Dress with squeezed lemon and black pepper.

TUNA BAGUETTE

Made with small (preferably wholemeal) baguette (about 3 oz), sliced lengthways and filled with 2 oz tuna in brine, drained and mixed with 1 teaspoon reduced-calorie mayonnaise. On top of tuna place lettuce, slices of pepper, tomato, cucumber and a little spring onion, if liked.

BIT OF EVERYTHING SALAD

Big bowl of fresh salad, all chopped up. Include crunchy vegetables like courgettes and cabbage (red or white) sliced. Add 1 oz lean (no skin) cooked chicken cut into thin strips, 1 oz lean (fat removed) beef or ham cut into thin strips and 1 oz reduced-fat, hard cheese, cut into thin strips. Mix everything together and add a splash of oil-free dressing with herbs, or try a spoonful of Weight Watchers' low-fat *Yoghurt and Mixed Herb* or *Mild Mustard* dressing.

◆ ◆ ◆

13 THIN DAYS

Unlike the Fat Days' eating plan, Thin Days is all about those days where food really is the last thing on your mind. However, you know it isn't sensible to ignore mealtimes, and so you want a diet plan that allows you to eat less but still feel good. Well, that's exactly where the Thin Days' diet can help.

You'll see that treats are kept to a minimum – that's because I'm assuming that if you're following this plan, you're too busy to think about them! And if you can manage to do without treats altogether, so much the better . . .

MIXING 'N' MATCHING

If you want to swap any of the breakfasts with the ones listed in chapter 5 that's fine as, calorie for calorie, all breakfasts work out the same. The lunch/light meals given here are slightly lower in calories than those that are given in the lunches' chapter, so bear that in mind if you're thinking of mixing and matching. However, if you are looking for alternatives, the main meals given for Thin Days are roughly the same calorific value as the lunches/light meals in chapter 6.

THE SEVEN-DAY PLAN

THIN DAY ONE

Breakfast
Small glass of orange juice ◆ 1 slice of wholemeal toast, scraping of low-fat spread, if wished, plus topping from selection of following: little reduced-sugar jam, reduced-sugar marmalade, yeast extract (e.g.

Marmite, Vecon etc.) or scraping of peanut butter, cottage cheese, sliver of reduced-fat, hard cheese ◆ Tea or coffee

Lunch
Cottage Cheese Mountain*, 2 crispbreads, if wanted ◆ Piece of fruit or diet yoghurt ◆ Hot or cold drink

Main meal
Chicken and Peach Salad*, wholemeal roll ◆ Diet fromage frais or diet yoghurt

Treats
1 (if wanted)

THIN DAY TWO

Breakfast
2 Weetabix, or supermarket own brand, milk from allowance, plus a little chopped fruit ◆ Tea or coffee

Lunch
Danish Sandwiches* ◆ Hot or cold drink

Main meal
Scrambled eggs, made with 2 eggs, splash of skimmed milk. Grilled tomato, 1 slice wholemeal toast.

Treats
1 (if wanted)

THIN DAY THREE

Breakfast
Small carton plain, low-fat yoghurt, mixed with 2 dessertspoons of no-added-sugar muesli and ½ sliced banana ◆ Tea or coffee, milk taken from allowance.

Lunch
1 soft-boiled egg, 1 slice of wholemeal bread, scraping of low-fat

spread ◆ Piece of fruit or diet yoghurt or fromage frais ◆ Hot or cold drink

Main meal
Ready-prepared meal up to 300 calories (e.g. Weight Watchers, Healthy Options, Lean Cuisine, Shapers or supermarket own band)

Treats
1 (if wanted)

THIN DAY FOUR

Breakfast
Small glass of fruit juice ◆ 1 slice of wholemeal toast, scraping of low-fat spread, topping from choice listed in day one ◆ Tea or coffee, milk taken from allowance

Lunch
Vegetable Platter* plus 2 crispbreads, if liked ◆ Diet yoghurt or diet fromage frais

Dinner
Tarragon Trout* plus 4 oz cooked rice ◆ If wanted, dessert chosen from selection on page 69

Treats
1 (if wanted)

THIN DAY FIVE

Breakfast
½ grapefruit, 2 crispbreads with scraping of low-fat spread and 1 boiled egg ◆ Tea or coffee, milk taken from allowance

Lunch
Sandwich made with 2 oz cottage cheese and a little chopped fruit (e.g. kiwi, pineapple, peach) ◆ Hot or cold drink

Main meal
Small portion (leg or thigh) of Chicken Thyme* with masses of salad
◆ If wanted, dessert from choice given on page 69

Treats
1 (if wanted)

THIN DAY SIX

Breakfast
Small glass of orange juice ◆ 1 slice of wholemeal toast, with topping chosen from day one ◆ Tea or coffee, milk taken from
allowance

Lunch
4 oz prawns, mixed with lemon juice and black pepper, served on a
bed of shredded lettuce. Served with 4 triangles bread, made from 1
wholemeal slice. Scraping of low-fat spread, if wanted ◆ Hot or cold
drink

Main meal
Spanish Noodles* ◆ Select fruit-based dessert from pages 67–68

Treats
1 (if wanted)

THIN DAY SEVEN

Breakfast
Small glass of orange juice ◆ Bowl of mixed fruits with spoonful of
plain yoghurt ◆ Tea or coffee, milk from allowance

Lunch
Feta Filler*, plus 1 crispbread ◆ Hot or cold drink

Dinner
Small portion of Fish Surprise* served with 2 oz noodles or ready-
prepared meal (as listed on day three) ◆ If wanted, dessert from
choice given on page 69, or a piece of fruit

Treats
1 (if wanted)

RECIPES

COTTAGE CHEESE MOUNTAIN

As much salad as you can manage, roughly chopped, and served in
large bowl. Pile high with 4 oz creamy, reduced-fat cottage cheese.
Top with half a dozen bite-sized pieces of pineapple (either fresh, or
pineapple pieces canned in fruit juice).

SPINACH NOODLES

little oil
2 onions, sliced
2 cloves garlic, chopped small
8 oz cooked spinach, either fresh or frozen
black pepper
1 teaspoon mixed herbs
½ teaspoon nutmeg
sprinkling of Parmesan, to serve

Brush non-stick pan with little oil, then cook onion and garlic for
5–10 minutes, until onion becomes transparent, stirring all the time.
Chop spinach roughly (be sure to squeeze out excess water if using
recently-defrosted frozen). Add spinach to pan, mixing well. Add seasoning and continue to cook, on a low heat for 10 minutes or so, until
spinach is cooked through. Add 4 oz cooked noodles, per person. Toss
well and place in serving dish. Sprinkle with Parmesan and serve.

FETA FILLER

Use lots of crunchy lettuce, cucumber, sliced thinly, stoned unstuffed
olives, plus 2 oz Feta cheese, cut into small chunks. Add a splash of
oil-free dressing with herbs, or, if preferred, add fresh dill and a good
squeeze of lemon juice.

VEGETABLE PLATTER

As many raw vegetables as you can bear to stand and wash, peel and scrape (choose from peppers, celery, courgettes, mini corns, cucumber) cut into thick sticks, about 2 inches long, plus cauliflower and broccoli florets, served with selection of low-fat, low-calorie dips, either bought from the supermarket ready prepared or home-made using: 1 oz reduced-calorie mayonnaise, squeeze of lemon juice and pinch of curry powder, 2 oz low-fat, soft cheese, ½ – 1 crushed garlic clove (depending on your taste), ½ teaspoon fresh herbs. Or serve with 1 oz virtually fat-free fromage frais, mixed with 1 crushed garlic clove and 1 teaspoon tomato purée.

VEGETABLE KEBABS

On kebab skewers, thread mushrooms (if large ones, cut in half), slices of courgette, tomato and chunks of pepper, sweetcorn, shallots, or small onions – and whatever else is threadable! Place on grill pan, brush lightly with mixture of oil and lemon juice and grill for around 10 minutes. Turn kebabs regularly to avoid burning on one side. Serve with 6 oz cooked rice or pasta.

DANISH SANDWICHES

Take 2 small slices of pumpernickel bread, scraped with low-fat spread. Cover one with 1 oz smoked turkey, topped with slices of tomato, cucumber and gherkin, the other with 1 oz pastrami, topped with slices of tomato, cucumber and gherkin.

CHICKEN AND PEACH SALAD

Mix 3 oz cooked chicken (skin removed), thinly sliced with 2 oz tinned peaches, canned in own juice, thinly sliced. Place on a bed of crunchy lettuce, thinly sliced cucumber and watercress. Dress with lime juice, a splash of oil-free dressing or 1 tablespoon peach juice. This is wonderful with a fresh peach or fresh mango, if in season.

For recipes for soups and desserts, turn to chapter 7.

◆ ◆ ◆

14 EXERCISE

When I first sat down to write this book, I have to admit that I had no intention whatsoever of including anything but the bare minimum on exercise. My feeling was that this was to be a *diet* book and exercise had absolutely no place in a diet book – if anyone wanted to read about the best way to writhe around in a leotard, I reasoned, then they could buy an *exercise* book. There was no way I was going to bore my readers with pages on sports centres and trendy fitness clubs, finding the 'right sort of trainer', or advice on how to turn your lounge into your own personal gym.

As you can probably detect, 'exercise' is not my favourite word and I've almost been proud of the fact that, until recently, I had *never* been to an exercise class, never bought an exercise tape and didn't possess a leotard. 'Going for the burn' only ever happened to me when I got too near the stove, while 'warming up' was something that was felt only after a good five minutes soaking in a steaming, hot bath. For me, workouts were made up of groups of eccentrics who seemed to enjoy getting their bodies into positions that I considered obscene, impossible or certifiable. In fact, having witnessed several classes up close, I have to admit this was most definitely not my idea of fun. However, much as I may have scoured the medical press and health surveys, there seemed little to support my idle ways.

Reluctantly, and I suppose even begrudgingly, I have to admit that all the medical evidence is unequivocal – exercise *is* good for just about everyone – and to be a successful slimmer, moving more is almost as important as eating less. In fact, there are some experts who believe that slimmers have been too concerned about what they eat and not concerned enough with what they do. That said, for all those who want to read about exercise even less than they want to do it, I promise to get the rest of this chapter over with quickly!

As we've already seen in chapter 2, exercise generally helps speed up the metabolic rate (the rate you burn calories) but the good news is that the right sort of exercise can mean that you continue burning off calories at a higher rate for some time after the actual exercising has stopped; the effect can last up to 24 hours. So, you not only lose weight faster, but after a bout of exercise you continue burning up calories, even when you're doing nothing!

Also, the more emphasis there is in your life on exercise, or your *output*, the less emphasis there need be on your *input* (the actual amount you eat) because, if you balance things right, your increased output should be able to 'mop-up' any excessive input. And, of course, the more exercise you do, the less chance you actually have to eat anything, whether you want to or not! And once you've taken your mind off food, you're halfway there to winning the weight battle.

You might also be interested to know that exercise has been scientifically shown to actually act as a supressant to the appetite, as it helps prevent a drop in the blood sugar levels which give rise to hunger; it's when your blood sugar level drops that you feel hungry and regular exercise stabilises the blood sugar level.

Of course if you're unhappy with your body – and would you be buying a diet book if you weren't? – then you're probably not feeling all that inclined to exercise in the first place. But, however much you may hate even the thought of any physical activity, in the long term it can make day-to-day living an awful lot easier, and that's apart from helping you slim.

So, if ever you've found it difficult to get up from the floor (or down there in the first place) or you've found you're exhausted after running for the bus, playing in the garden with the children, or even after carrying the bags back from the supermarket, then that should give you enough motivation to at least give exercise a try. Regular exercise means you'll be fitter and have more energy to do the things that you enjoy doing; get the balance right, and you should find that you'll be able to eat more *without* putting on any weight.

◆ GOING GREEN

Exercise is also excellent for toning up muscles, as well as helping to reduce fat. This is because exercise increases the lean tissue in the body, while at the same time reducing the fat tissue. As any well-seasoned slimmer knows, regardless of how strict your slimming regime is, unless you indulge in at least some exercise a couple of times a week the rolls just seem to get saggier, rather than tighter.

When we're young, fitness seems to come almost naturally; we spend much of the time tearing around almost impervious to fatigue. And as youngsters, our bodies are also seemingly devoid of wear and tear. But, the older we get, the more likely we are to do the bare minimum. It may be because we're in a hurry (isn't the car so much quicker than walking?) or we're in the habit; whatever the reason, we seem to have all but programmed our bodies to do as little as possible. Maybe it's a way of making our bodies environmentally sound – rather than make any unnecessary moves, we prefer to conserve our energy.

The reality is, though, that if we don't make full use of our bodies, they start to deteriorate. Our muscles end up considerably weaker and softer and our circulation becomes sluggish. It's a bit like a car – if you don't keep your engine finely tuned, pretty soon you're going to need a re-fit. No wonder tight, firm muscles are the preserve of the very young, well preserved or well exercised! However, the good news is that along with a sensible eating plan, when you exercise the muscles become more elastic, the fat you're storing decreases and, amazingly, you'll find that your body starts to reclaim its old shape.

Saying that exercise can help keep you alive may seem far fetched but there's an awful lot of evidence to suggest that taking part in regular physical activity can reduce our risk of a number of major diseases. It strengthens our heart, improves our circulation, increases the capacity as well as efficiency of our lungs, relieves stress, keeps us supple and, particularly important for women, it helps increase bone-density which means it offers protection against the bone-thinning disease, *osteoporosis*, which causes bones to become brittle and so fracture more easily.

And if you're still not convinced, there's the feel good factor to consider – and that's official. Exercise stimulates the release of *endorphins*, the body's natural pain-killers, which produces a general feeling of well-being. So much so, that some doctors have recommended exercise to help alleviate depression as well as insomnia. And it's been shown to be more effective at fighting anti-ageing effects on your body than many of the pills and potions you can buy over the counter – and it's an awful lot cheaper!

So what's the least you can get away with?

Now, if like me, you're a slow convert to believing there's anything positive to say about physical activity, then you're probably keen to know how little you need to do before you can reap all these wonderful physical as well as mental benefits. Well, in a sentence, the minimum you should be aiming for is 20–30 minutes vigorous exercise, at least three times a week.

There are two different types of exercise: *aerobic* such as jogging, swimming, cycling etc. and *anaerobic*. Anaerobic exercises are those that consist of short, sharp bursts of muscle activity, such as tennis and squash. The secret is to make sure all your exercises are aerobic ones which work all the large muscle groups (like those found in the legs and trunk), plus the heart, lungs and circulatory system, as well as burning up calories. For the exercise to be really beneficial, you need to do it vigorously – enough to get you huffing and puffing. The idea is that you should still be able to have a conversation after a session of aerobic exercise, albeit a slightly breathless one. So, it's the continuous exercises that you need to opt for, like swimming, jogging, running, cycling, walking briskly – even dancing or skipping. You need something where you're 'on the go' all the time, although breaking exercising into 12-minute bouts might be easier to handle, both mentally as well as physically!

Picking the exercise to fit your style

If you have decided that you are going to give exercise a try, you obiously want to do something that helps your weight, as well as your shape, so below is a choice of what's available, with some advice on how to get started. And as with choosing the diets to suit your mood, there's nothing to stop you mixing and matching your exercises. So, you may decide to swim once a week but spend your other 30-minute blocks of exercise walking, or even at an organised exercise class. It's up to you. No-one says you have to lock yourself into, say, jogging three times a week, all alone when you'd rather do something that the rest of the family can join in. The idea is that you should enjoy the increased physical activity, so spending time doing what you *want* to do, rather than what you think you *ought* to do, is bound to be more effective for your body as well as your mind. The more you enjoy it, the more chance there is that you'll stick with it.

WALKING

You may not think of walking as *real* exercise but it is. In fact, if you walk an extra mile every day for a year, you could lose 10 lb – and that's without dieting! Walking is recommended as a good starting point for the type of person who rarely exercises and probably can't even remember the last time they exerted themselves! This is certainly one of the easiest ways to get into shape because you can fit it in whenever you have the time. You don't need to worry about booking classes or special clothes – it's all down to you. That said, a gentle stroll down your local high street is *not* considered exercise. For walking to have any effect, you need to aim to walk briskly, arms swinging as you go, for 20–30 minutes without stopping, at least three times a week. If you are unfit though, you're best to limit yourself to 5–10 minutes of brisk walking to begin with. Don't push yourself so that you end up feeling uncomfortable or too exhausted to walk back home. That's not the aim of the exercise!

SWIMMING

Swimming is probably one of the best all-round activities, particularly if you're overweight, as the water supports your body. Most pools are open a variety of hours, so you can usually fit in a visit to suit you, be it lunch time, first thing in the morning or in the evening. Check local pools for details. Ultimately you want to aim for 20–30 minutes non-stop swimming but you should build this up slowly, particularly if you're not used to exercise. Swimming can also be particularly tiring so don't push yourself too hard; gentle swimming (any stroke you like) is fine to start with, until you feel fit enough to build up to something more vigorous.

Jogging/Running

Like walking, running or jogging – a gentle sort of running – is cheap (although it's important to invest in a good pair of running shoes) and you can run when and where you want to. It's a very good exercise for both your heart and lungs and it's easy enough to pace yourself so that you stop when you feel your body has had enough. You also don't need to jog alone, so try nagging an equally unfit friend to join you. If you do like the idea of jogging, or running, and you're relatively new to the exercise game, experts recommend that you start walking first and then build up to a jog.

Cycling

Some people prefer an exercise bike to the real thing and although you could miss out on fresh air and picturesque scenery, if you live near a main road in a busy town, the inside version of cycling may actually do your sensibilities, as well as your lungs less harm! Obviously the easiest way of working cycling into your lifestyle is to cycle everywhere but the practicalities of doing this depend on where you live. Outdoor cycling can be an activity the whole family can share but if you're not sure it's for you, then before you splash out on the latest model, or even a second-hand one, try borrowing a bike for a week or so. As with other forms of exercise, if you're a novice don't push yourself too hard to begin with; start slowly and build up to longer and more frequent sessions, getting your legs to work harder as you get more proficient. If you've opted for an exercise bike, once again build up slowly, although most machines can easily be adjusted so that you set yourself ever increasing targets.

Aerobic exercise/dance classes

These are organised classes where the aim of the session is to swiftly move from one set of exercises to another, without stopping, in time to music. It's vital that your teacher is qualified so that she knows what she's doing; attempting an exercise that is beyond your level of fitness can be dangerous, as well as painful. As with other aerobic exercises, you need to feel you're getting relatively breathless after a short session (many classes are simply based on stretching which, while excellent for stamina and suppleness, are not *aerobic*). With any classes, ensure that you have a 5–10 minute warm up and cool down period which allows your body to adjust to the sharp change in pace. A good teacher will keep a watch on beginners and will usually suggest that you do whatever exercises you can; no-one expects you to keep up when you've never done it before! It's also important to make sure you don't push yourself. The idea is not to be flat on your back from exhaustion within five minutes of starting – remember, the aim is to be slightly out of breath, not totally breathless. And the most important rule is that if it hurts, stop *immediately*. Ask around for details of local classes or at the library or your local adult education centre.

SKIPPING

Yes, that old playground favourite offers a wonderful opportunity for cheap and convenient exercise, right on your doorstep. To be really effective you have to work up to around 20 minutes of skipping but if you get bored, there's nothing to stop you breaking off for a few minutes running on the spot. Once again, start slowly and gently, and gradually build up your time.

. . . AND THE REST

Activities such as tennis and squash are excellent when it comes to overall fitness but as they involve a lot of stopping and starting they can be hard to maintain for any length of time without a break. So, strictly speaking, unless you have the stamina of Bjorn Borg, the chances are you won't be exercising aerobically. And if you are overweight and unused to exercise of any sort, all these sports can put quite a strain on the uninitiated. In fact, you need to be fairly fit in the first place just to sustain a game in any of these sports. However, all the activities will certainly increase your overall fitness level, which is no bad thing.

There are then exercises like weight-training on offer. These will certainly improve your overall strength but although they will get you huffing and puffing, they're not aerobic. Remember, their aim is to build up particular muscles, rather than building up your heart and lungs. The same is true of exercises like isometrics, which are based on increasing muscle strength. So, if you really want to lose it, you're going to have to move it and 'it' refers to the whole body, not just part of it!

GOING IT ALONE

Of course you don't need to join a class to take part in an organised aerobic session. You may well find it more convenient, and, come to that, less embarrassing, to exercise in the privacy of your own home along with a video, or sound tape, for guidance. Tapes are available at most high street stores, as well as newsagents, but whichever one you buy, make sure that the exercises have been put together by a qualified expert who knows what they're doing, or, more accurately, what they're getting you to do. At certain times of the year the shops are hit by a rash of 'celebrity' tapes and while some might be safe-and-sound, others are decidedly dodgy, so do choose carefully. It's also important to make sure that you choose a tape that offers exercises that are at the right level for you. If you really are a beginner, buy a beginners' tape; anything more advanced won't make you fitter, it'll just make you depressed because you won't be able to keep up. There's no point in buying advanced aerobics when you haven't even reached first base! And if you don't like the idea of disembodied voices giving you instructions but you *do* like dancing, what about digging out some old records and dancing to them?

BEING SAFE RATHER THAN SORRY

A word of warning! If you're unfit or unused to exercise it's important to remember that aerobic exeriqse should be built up *slowly*. If you're unfit, your muscles are short of oxygen and you won't get an adequate supply when you exercise. To be on the safe side, if you really are unused to being active and you still have quite a bit of weight to lose, check with your doctor before you undertake any regular exercise, particularly if your new-found enthusiasm ends up making you undertake a schedule which, prior to this diet, would have produced a glazed expression and a quick retreat!

And if you have high blood pressure, a heart condition, or suffer with asthma or arthritis, you *must* talk to your doctor before undertaking anything which might be a little too gruelling for you – a more appropriate activity may be recommended. The same applies if you've recently had an operation; recovery time from any operation or illness depends on what the surgery was for, so it's always best to be on the safe side by having a word with your doctor before starting any new, vigorous activity.

Whatever your state of health, it's always important to start with relatively gentle exercises, then build up to something more strenuous as you get more active – for example, swimming or walking. Whatever you choose, it's important to spend at least five minutes at the beginning and at the end of each session with gentle, stretching routines (the infamous *warming up* and *winding/cooling down*), as this gradually increases the supply of energy to your muscles, ensuring that they work at their best, and avoids the chance of damage, such as a tear or strain; they also help reduce after-class stiffness, the following day. Warming up releases tension in the muscles and stretches them out, getting them ready for exercising.

If you are new to the exercise game it's often worth joining some organised group or class run by a qualified instructor. That way you can be sure that the amount of physical acitivity you're undertaking is the right level for you and that all the exercises, whether warmups or press-ups, are properly supervised. If you don't feel happy with the idea of going to something organised, or simply can't fit it into your day then it's worth trying a video or sound tape (see Going It Alone, on the opposite page).

Whichever exercise you decide to opt for, it's worth remembering that those three half-hour sessions should be something you look forward to. So, choose something that you at least think you might enjoy. If you've always thought the idea of physical activity boring, try to find someone to exercise with, whether that means going to organised classes, sports centres or going for a run. It really doesn't matter. The important thing is to make sure you enjoy it; that way you'll keep on going. And, if in the meantime, your exercise sessions become an important part of your social life – so what? At least it means you're less likely to lose interest!

AND EXERCISE FOR THOSE THAT DON'T

If the whole idea of exercise really does make you want to lie down in a darkened room, then you should at least be looking at less obtrusive ways of boosting your activity level. If you at least *try* to aim to follow some of the ideas below then at least it will get you moving. And as long as you remember that when it comes to weight, you really do have to move to lose, then all you have to do is decide how much you really want to lose and move accordingly!

- ◆ Always, always, use the stairs rather than the lift. The only time you have an excuse is if you have a buggy/baby with you!
- ◆ Everytime you go up the stairs at home try running up them.
- ◆ If you've taken the car (are you sure you couldn't have walked or taken the bus so *some* walking would be involved?) and you're parking in a car park, leave the car as far away from the entrance as possible.
- ◆ If you've only a short journey to make, don't wait for the bus, walk. You'll probably get there quicker anyway.
- ◆ Get into the habit of taking a dog for a walk. Puppies are best as they move quickly and can keep going for ages. If you don't have a dog, don't you know someone who does?
- ◆ If there's music on the radio, and you're at home, dance.
- ◆ Offer to play chase with the kids.
- ◆ Hide all remote control boxes.
- ◆ If you do have to walk anywhere, make sure you do it briskly, striding out, arms swinging to and fro.
- ◆ Think before you sink – whether it's into your car, an armchair, a park bench – could you be doing something to help burn up some of that excess fat?

The more you get into the habit of using your body, the greater the difference it will make to your overall energy output. And the greater your output, the nearer you get to your goal. And isn't that what reading a diet book is about?

◆ ◆ ◆

15 PULLING IN YOUR BELT

This is the chapter aimed specifically at those of you who will be doing just that because as a new, slimmer you, your clothes are now so loose that if you don't wear a belt, they'll look much too big!

If you're reading this and *have* reached you goal weight then well done – you have every right to be exceedingly proud of yourself! Now you've just got to make sure that, give or take a little, your weight doesn't start to waiver. As I hope you've seen, it shouldn't be difficult to maintain your goal and there's no reason why your lifestyle should suffer just because you want to stay the same size. Of course there are days when you may over-indulge but, now armed with your new, nutritional know-how, at least you'll be aware of what you've done, which means you can compensate for any excesses by being careful what you eat the next day.

Maintaining your weight at the level you feel happy with really is all about recognising what is a good diet – and a bad one. For many women the problem of sticking to the right sort of diet depends not on what they cook, but how they cook it. The recipes included in this book have, I hope, at least given you the flavour of cooking for a slimmer you. While I've tried to make the recipes varied so that they suit all different tastes, you may well want to adapt them to suit yourself and your family. However, on the following pages are some basic ground rules which I hope will be helpful in keeping your cooking low on fat but high on taste.

If you enjoy cooking and are looking for new low-fat and low-calorie ideas, it's worth looking at some of the recipes in magazines. Many have recipes which are specifically devised for those who are watching their weight and most publications give a nutritional analysis of the meals they've devised so you can see, at-a-glance, how many calories each dish contains per serving.

However, if you're more interested in adapting *your* recipes rather than trying out new ones, by following a few simple rules, it is still possible to gain on taste, vitamins and minerals – the only thing you're really likely to lose out on is calories, and the beauty of it is, you haven't even had to think about it!

SO, WHEN YOU'RE SHOPPING

- Choose lean cuts of meat
- Buy skimmed milk, low-fat and reduced-sugar products
- If you're buying tinned fruit or vegetables, make sure they're in their own juice or canned in water
- Avoid all supermarket aisles containing biscuits, cakes, chocolates, pies, pastries, nuts, crisps
- Where possible, avoid meat products such as pies, pasties, sausages, burgers
- Try to avoid processed foods – most have fats, sugar and salt added, all of which you can do without
- If you're buying fizzy drinks or squashes, make sure they are either no- or low-calorie

WHEN YOU'RE COOKING

- Where possible, grill and baste with lemon juice. If you find the food is drying out use a pastry brush to lightly cover with a little polyunsaturated oil
- Try baking, poaching or microwaving
- If you have to fry, use a non-stick pan. If you don't possess one just dip a pastry brush in a little 'light' polyunsaturated oil and then coat the pan thinly. Before serving food, pat on a little kitchen roll as this will absorb any excess oil
- When you're cooking meat, remember to trim off all visible fat
- Where appropriate, drain pan of all meat fat before adding other ingredients
- Don't forget to remove skin from poultry
- If you're roasting, try using a trivet or a rack so that the fat drips into the pan. Cover food with foil or greaseproof paper and baste regularly so meat doesn't dry out
- If you're making a casserole, do it a day ahead. You'll find that, when cold, the fat will float to the top of the saucepan so you can simply skim it off

- Use a steamer (a metal colander will do) whenever possible. Steaming really does bring out the natural flavour of foods, particularly vegetables, and that's without adding a thing!
- If you like your gravy, then buy yourself a gravy boat or jug that has a spout with a built-in strainer which catches the fat
- Thicken casseroles and soups with puréed vegetables, yoghurt or fromage frais. Make sauces with cornflour

And for those of you who prefer to think about what you can eat, rather than what you can't:

- Eat *more* fish, lean meat and poultry
- Eat *more* pulses (like beans, peas, and lentils)
- Eat *more* fresh fruit and vegetables
- Eat *more* wholemeal pasta, wholemeal bread and brown rice
- Drink *as much* water as you like

▼HOSE HIDDEN EXTRAS

It also helps if you get into the habit of looking at labels so that you become familiar with all those extra ingredients that manufacturers add. They're listed in descending order of quantities so if sugar, or indeed fat, is one of the top three ingredients put the food back on the shelf! If you feel it really is something that you *must* have then eat sparingly or reserve it for a special occasion.

It also pays to know the various names that manufacturers can use for a fairly standard product. *Sugar*, for example, is a term used for several different things, such as: honey, syrup, treacle, molasses or glucose syrups. Also manufactured sugars, found in our packaged foods, could be listed as: *sucrose, lactose, dextrose, maltose, glucose* or *fructose*. So be warned! And, if you think you only need to look at the labels of 'sweet' foods, you're mistaken. A small tin of tomato soup could contain up to three teaspoons of sugar, tomato ketchup has around a tablespoon of the stuff, while a couple of ounces of muesli may well have up to three teaspoons added to it.

Also beware of food that's loaded with hidden fat. Biggest offenders are: sausages, luncheon meats, liver sausage, many pâtés, salami and meat pies. And go easy on eggs. One egg contains the equivalent of a teaspoon of fat!

And one other word of advice. Read the labels *before* you buy – don't wait until you get home!

AND LASTLY...

Well, now you're a successful slimmer you know exactly how easy it is to diet in a way that suits your lifestyle as well as your mood. Having lost your excess weight you no longer need to worry about following a slim plan to the letter. Just understanding some of the basic rules about cooking – and eating – should be enough to keep you at your goal weight.

It's worth remembering, though, that staying slim on this slim plan isn't about denying yourself food or encouraging you to feel heaps of guilt everytime you're in touching distance of a chocolate bar! A little of what you fancy often really does do you good, as long as it is a little, and not too often. One small portion of chocolate mousse won't hurt but three bowlfuls will.

And if you do find your weight creeping up the scales, albeit ever so slowly, there's no need to panic – or comfort eat for that matter! All you do is go on a quick seven-day fat blitz: just decide on the type of week you have ahead (whether you're likely to be at home or relying on fast foods as you dash around the place) and choose the appropriate seven-day slim plan. It really couldn't be easier. Remember, all it takes is just *7 Days to a Slimmer You* . . .

◆ ◆ ◆

RECORDING SUCCESS

YOUR TARGET LOSS

At the end of week one _____

At the end of week two _____

At the end of week three _____

At the end of week four _____

At the end of week five _____

At the end of week six _____

At the end of week seven _____

weight loss	week one	week two	week three	week four	week five	week six	week seven
14lb							
13lb							
12lb							
11lb							
10lb							
9lb							
8lb							
7lb							
6lb							
5lb							
4lb							
3lb							
2lb							
1lb							

Plot your weight loss on this graph.

METRIC CONVERSION TABLE

	Approx. equivalent	Exact equivalent
¼ oz	5 g	7.0 g
½ oz	10 g	14.1 g
1 oz	25 g	28.3 g
2 oz	50 g	56.6 g
3 oz	75 g	84.9 g
4 oz	100 g	113.2 g
5 oz	125 g	141.5 g
6 oz	150 g	169.8 g
7 oz	175 g	198.1 g
8 oz	200 g	227.0 g
9 oz	225 g	255.3 g
10 oz	250 g	283.0 g
11 oz	275 g	311.3 g
12 oz	300 g	340.0 g
13 oz	325 g	368.3 g
14 oz	350 g	396.6 g
15 oz	375 g	424.0 g
16 oz	400 g	454.0 g
2 lb	1 kg	908.0 g
¼ pt	125 ml	142 ml
½ pt	250 ml (¼ litre)	284 ml
¾ pt	375 ml	426 ml
1 pt	500 ml (½ litre)	568 ml
1½ pt	750 ml (¾ litre)	852 ml
2 pt (1 qt)	1000 ml (1 litre)	1.13 litre